DIET
AND
DOMESTIC
LIFE IN
SOCIETY

DIET
AND
DOMESTIC
LIFE IN
SOCIETY

EDITED BY

Anne Sharman

Janet Theophano

Karen Curtis

Ellen Messer

Temple University Press

Philadelphia

Temple University Press, Philadelphia 19122
Copyright © 1991 by Temple University. All rights reserved
Published 1991
Printed in the United States of America

The paper used in this publication meets the minimum
requirements of American National Standard for Information
Sciences—Permanence of Paper for Printed Library Materials,
ANSI Z39.49-1984 ∞

Library of Congress Cataloging-in-Publication Data

Diet and domestic life in society / edited by Anne Sharman . . . [et
al.].
        p.   cm.
    Based on the symposium "Diet and Domestic Organization,"
held at the American Anthropological Association Annual
Meeting, Dec. 1981, in Los Angeles, Calif.
    Includes bibliographical references and index.
    ISBN 0-87722-751-9
    1. Food habits—Cross-cultural studies—Congresses.
2. Nutrition—Cross-cultural studies—Congresses.   3. Home
economics—Cross-cultural studies—Congresses.   I. Sharman,
Anne, 1940–
II. American Anthropological Association. Meeting (1981 : Los
Angeles, Calif.)
GT2850.D52   1991
394.1′2—dc20   90-40636
                                                    CIP

Contents

Acknowledgments

This book has grown out of a symposium on diet and domestic organization held at the American Anthropological Association Annual Meeting, December 1981, in Los Angeles, California. During its long gestation period many people have given generously of their time, ideas, and support. We wish to thank them all, and especially Anna Lou Dehavenon, Anne Fleuret, Judith Goode, Thomas Marchione, Michael Murtaugh, and Meredith Turshen.

The editors owe a special debt to the constructive involvement and patience of the other contributors and to Jane Cullen and Deborah Stuart at Temple University Press. The skill and generosity of Nadia Kravchenko, who word processed the manuscript in its various forms, made that difficult task appear easy.

DIET
AND
DOMESTIC
LIFE IN
SOCIETY

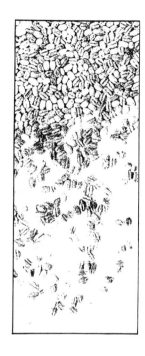

Introduction

Anne Sharman

Janet Theophano

Karen Curtis

Ellen Messer

This book explores the importance of domestic life for understanding dietary practices and the distribution of nutritional status. All contributors are anthropologists who share certain general orientations. Together they present a general approach to analyzing diet and domestic life in society based on recent trends in anthropology, and a view of the contribution anthropology can make in formulating, implementing, and evaluating food and nutrition policy.

In most societies the greater part of people's eating takes place in a domestic context, and it is frequently here that choices about diet and use of resources are made, even when people subsequently eat outside the domestic sphere. Domestic units are generally important centers of biological and social reproduction, where children are nurtured, fed, and taught and where, throughout their lives, people continue to learn and to redefine their dietary ideas and practices in relation to their changing circumstances and experiences.

In the study of domestic processes it can be seen how and why large-scale organization (at local, regional, national, and international levels) and systems of social stratification (and consequently people's cultural, social, economic, and political positions) affect diet and nutrition. It can be seen how at a microlevel mechanisms operate that at all levels contribute to impoverishing and malnourishing some people and sections of populations and promoting the relative well-being of others. The success or failure of important aspects of food and nutrition programs may also rest on the dynamics of domestic organization (Rogers 1983).

Yet before the early 1980s few anthropologists had carried out research focused on the relation between domestic life, food, and nutrition (Messer 1983). In attempting to understand patterns of food consumption and nutritional status, they tended (with exceptions) to focus more generally on cultural patterns and on aspects of the social and economic organization of whole societies. In doing so, they also tended to emphasize patterns shared by members of particular cultures and societies and thus to stress homogeneity rather than variability (Montgomery 1978). In food and nutritional

4

anthropology the shift in interest that occurred in the early 1980s reflected both changes in theoretical orientations and concern with practical issues confronting those involved in food and nutrition planning.

This introduction outlines the general approach shared by contributors and discusses its significance for the analysis of diet and domestic life in society. It also points out the relevance of this approach to food and nutrition policy. Chapter 11 (Sharman, Theophano, Curtis, and Messer) suggests some directions for further research and looks in more detail at the policy implications of the point of view and data presented.

AN APPROACH TO THE STUDY OF DIETARY PRACTICES

> I also suggested that one could find scattered over the landscape the elements of a new trend that seems to be gathering force and coherence. . . . For the past several years, there has been growing interest in analysis focused through one or another of a bundle of interrelated terms: practice, praxis, action, interaction, activity, experience, performance. A second, and closely related, bundle of terms focuses on the doer of all that doing: agent, actor, person, self, individual, subject. (Ortner 1984, 144)

All contributors to this volume focus on small-scale activities and processes at the local level, as these generate and contribute to dietary practices. They see analysis of what people actually do as important in, and in many cases central to, their research. What people do is not seen primarily as the raw material from which can be abstracted cultural patterns (for example, cultural food habits) and social structure (for example, the structure of domestic groups in the society), but as the phenomenon that is to be analyzed and understood. People are seen as active in conducting their lives: as making choices and decisions, following strategies, negotiating, and improvising, so that their perceptions, points of view, and experience are considered critical for understanding the activities that researchers observe.

This general approach comprises an orientation rather than a unified theoretical framework. Reflecting the diverse strands of which it is composed, the contributors to this book draw on a range of different traditions in anthropology, and are all to some extent eclectic in developing their own particular approach. Some authors cite British functional and social structural antecedents, others those of American psychological and cultural anthropology. They variously make use of cognitive, symbolic (including semiotic), ecological, and marxist analyses, as well as others dealing more directly with practice, experience, interaction, and decision making (Ortiz, Chapter 10). The ethnographic case studies in this book suggest the richness and possibilities of this diversified approach for studying various aspects of diet and domestic life in society.

Part of the importance of such a perspective lies in the possibilities it provides for more flexible, open, and dynamic ways of analyzing interrelated cultural, social, economic, and political processes in relation to domestic life and diet. It presents ways of exploring the complexity and variability of social situations and people's circumstances, the practicalities of their lives, as these bear on dietary practices. Key ideas used by contributors include variability, informality,[1] process, time, context, and situation, together with various elements of the cluster of concepts focusing on people and how they conduct and arrange their lives. Such an approach takes into account people's distinct identities and interests, and evaluates, rather than presupposes, consensus, cooperation (which may occur without consensus), or conflict in social relationships. Ultimately it points to ways to integrate different levels of social analysis (Appadurai, Chapter 9). The rest of this section outlines how this general approach has facilitated more flexible and dynamic ways of analyzing culture, political economy and ecology, and domestic life in relation to dietary practices.

Culture

The way in which culture (and its relation to behavior and practice) is conceptualized in this general approach is different from some earlier formulations, such as that used in the cultural food habits approach (Mead 1943, 1949). The focus in analyzing cultural food habits was on group organization. Culture was analyzed as a unified system of ideas, beliefs, values, norms, and rules shared by group members and was considered to be the main determinant of dietary patterns. Even when this approach was modified to include a wider range of material and economic factors in analyzing dietary patterns, the view of culture remained a uniform and basically prescriptive one.

More recently, and in line with the emphasis on people as creative and active in conducting their lives, culture has been analyzed more as providing parameters within which people act, repertoires on which they draw, and means by which they communicate than as a system of beliefs, values, norms, and rules that prescribe their behavior. Cultural evaluations are seen as pervasive—an integral part of all perceptions, practices, and relationships—but also as variable and negotiable (Theophano and Curtis, Chapter 7). To quote from two anthropologists who have made important contributions to food and nutritional anthropology:

> The cognitive activity of the real life individual is largely devoted to building culture, patching it here and trimming it there, according to the exigencies of the day. In his very negotiating activity, each is forcing culture down the throats of his fellow men. When individuals transact, their medium of exchange is in units of culture. Their disputes are about standards and values. (Douglas 1978, 6)

> Although there remain strong tendencies among some anthropologists to argue polemically for and against attributing importance to beliefs in relation to people's interests and daily lives . . . , most contemporary anthropologists expect people to innovate, interpret, and rationalize their behavior, rather than

merely play out their roles according to a prepared cultural script. . . . The concept of behavioral flexibility in the face of ideology, however, is not current in many discussions of food behavior. (Laderman 1984, 547)

That a more uniform, rigid, controlling conception of culture and its relation to dietary patterns and behavior is still sometimes used by those formulating policy can have serious and detrimental implications for food and nutrition planning, as shown by Rizvi in Chapter 5.

Political Economy and Ecology

Analysis in terms of practice and those who do the practicing also makes possible more flexible and detailed analysis of people's variable use of the natural environment (where people still to some degree depend on agriculture, gardening, or gathering and hunting for food) and of the ways in which large-scale political and economic organization differentially defines their options and affects their social relationships (including domestic relationships), daily lives, and dietary practices. It emphasizes not only the major characteristics of the natural environment and the structure of the political economy, but also shows how small-scale variations in environment and circumstances, and a range of informal activities (carried out particularly by women and children), may have far-reaching effects on people's diet and nutritional status.

It further provides a way of looking at other kinds of complexities in the relationship between political economy and ecology, domestic life, and dietary practices. It makes it possible, for example, to trace the multiple paths by which large-scale organization affects people's diet and health (Scrimshaw and Cosminsky, Chapter 4) and the complex interrelations between women's activities and allocation of time, their income production and use, their domestic organization, and the diet and health of themselves and the members of their domestic units (Messer, Chapter 3).

Finally, it allows an open approach in identifying the spatial and social unit of study, since it is defined by tracing the activities and relationships relevant to the topic being considered. Children's foraging activities are confined to a small local area (Laderman, Chapter 2), but remittances as a source of income and food depend on migration and relationships that may cross international boundaries (Palacio, Chapter 6).

Domestic Life

Flexibility in defining units of study, made possible by focusing on activities, is also important in examining domestic life and diet within the context of the political economy. As already mentioned, women's (and children's and sometimes men's) performance of typically domestic activities is often closely interwoven with a range of other food-acquisition and income-generating tasks, so that the domestic domain is not a clearly discrete and separate one. In addition, in many societies food-related activities (acquisition, distribution, consumption, and associated storage and preparation) and other undertakings that affect the diet, nutrition, and health of domestic units and their members (such as child care, care of the sick, daily maintenance of the living space, and budgeting of cash) are not all carried out by the same group of people.

In an attempt to clarify their conceptualizations in thinking about domestic life, anthropologists have come to distinguish between domestic units defined primarily by kinship and marriage ("families"), units defined primarily by shared residence (including "households"), and groups organized around a range of domestic activities. Considerations of proximity, friendship, age, and shared interests (for example, religious), in addition to those of kinship and residence, may affect who participates with whom, when, and in what shared activities and may be the bases of recruitment for different activity groupings. Thus, it is often not possible or useful to draw distinct boundaries around *the* domestic unit. The relevant unit for dietary analyses in a society may be more inclusive, less inclusive, or simply different in different situations.

The fact that for the study of domestic activities, domestic resources, and diet there is often no single appropriate domestic unit in a society has been recognized for a long time (Sharman 1970a,

1970b); and recently Messer (1983) has discussed the full range of possible groupings that might be identified and be relevant to particular dietary investigations. At the same time, however, other anthropologists studying diet and nutrition continue to write as if there were one such domestic unit, the household, which could be universally identified and used for comparison between societies (Lieberman 1986). But in cases where households are an important unit of study, they are often part of larger residential units or tied into larger family or occupational groupings and are frequently open and flexible. Individuals may move freely between them, and activity groupings may cut across their boundaries. For purposes of eating, as well as sometimes budgeting and other activities, a number of subunits may be identifiable within households (Sharman, Chapter 8). Members may also have conflicting interests and do not necessarily form a unified group.

Food and nutritional anthropologists became particularly interested in studying domestic units when they started looking for explanations for variations in diet and nutrition found within the same society or culture, and even within the same domestic unit (Gross and Underwood 1971; Sharman 1970a, 1970b). At first, those who further explored the relation between domestic organization and dietary practices focused especially on the distribution of food within the household or family (Horowitz 1980; Marchione 1981; Pelto 1983; Van Esterik 1984). Now, more comprehensive analysis of the workings of, and relations between, domestic units is being emphasized (Rogers 1983; contributors to this book). This is also the case in the closely related area of economic anthropology (Rutz and Orlove 1989; Wilks 1989).

Detailed analysis is needed of the contributions women, men, and children of different ages and statuses make to the domestic economy and domestic life in different social situations and of the complexities of power, control, and influence within domestic units as these bear on decision making, acquisition and allocation of resources, and dietary practices. Again, it is important to understand not only the formal structure and organization of domestic units—who is supposed to control and do what—but also informal activities. Women are often finally responsible for seeing that the members of their domestic units are fed, but their access to and control over resources sometimes depends to a large extent on informal and ad hoc arrangements.

The general approach presented in this book suggests ways of looking at the complexities of domestic life as they bear on dietary practices and are related to larger scale organization. The contributions show some applications of the approach and the methods of data collection and analysis used.

CASE STUDIES AND ETHNOGRAPHY

Study of practice and of the perceptions, points of view, and experience of people active in conducting their lives—of the *processes* that link dietary practices, domestic life, and larger-scale organization—does not lend itself to quantitative analysis. It must depend to a large extent on collection and analysis of qualitative data and on participant observation and the use of case studies. All contributors make use of qualitative methods. Where quantitative methods of data collection are also used, interpretation of the results depends on qualitative data collected by other methods.

Ethnographic studies (firsthand descriptions and analyses of particular societies or cultures) are a form of case study. In presenting ethnographic material, other kinds of case studies, more limited in scale and of varying time span and depth, may also be used to convey information and to make general, theoretical points. In this volume, case studies used by contributors in presenting ethnographic data include what Gluckman (1961) has described as apt illustration, social situations, and extended case studies.

Analysis using a small number of case studies is often criticized on the grounds that there is no way of knowing whether the cases presented are typical of the population being studied. Particularly where case studies use largely qualitative rather than quantitative analysis, there is a tendency to see them as unscientific and as involving a lot of unnecessary detail and complexity. Mitchell (1983, 188) argues that such a view "betrays a confusion between procedures appropriate to making inferences from statistical data and those appropriate to the study of an idiosyncratic combination of elements which constitute a 'case.'"

He makes a distinction between statistical inference on the one hand and logical/scientific/causal inference on the other. The latter is necessary for interpreting statistical relationships, and case-study analysis, when rigorously conducted, is particularly useful in developing this kind of thinking. He further argues:

1. The case study contrasts with "the 'survey' type of analysis, in which the person is replaced by the trait as the unit of analysis" (192)
2. Almost all case studies include consideration of processes and of developments in the phenomena being studied
3. The breadth of data included in case-study analysis is an important part of the approach. The rich detail that emerges from the intimate knowledge the analyst must acquire in a case study if it is well-conducted provides the optimum conditions for the acquisition of those illuminating insights that make formerly opaque connections suddenly pellucid (207). In this it is akin to Geertz's (1973) advocacy of "thick description" for understanding the meaning of what people do.

It is these characteristics of case study analysis that make it important in exploring critical issues in the study of dietary practices and domestic life in society.

FOOD AND NUTRITION POLICY

The need to be able to specify more precisely the processes that lead to particular patterns of food use and nutritional status and the related need to understand more clearly what goes on within domestic units are recurring themes in discussing food and nutrition policy. It is necessary to know not only what factors, including programs, affect diet and nutrition, but also how, why, to what extent, and in what context they do so.

Such information is often not generated by the research designs, and survey and other techniques, used by nutritionists, economists, and others involved with food and nutrition issues. The approach in this book offers a way of looking at diet and domestic life in society that can generate additional kinds of information necessary as a basis for formulating, implementing, and evaluating food and nutrition policies and programs.

NOTE

1. Formal and informal are relative terms, whose precise meaning can vary with the situation. In writing about domestic organization, formal usually refers to generally accepted ideals and rules that define preferred residence, division of labor, and rights and obligations between members of domestic units. In relation to the economy, formal often denotes the main productive enterprises in an area and the legal rules regulating their operation. Informal economic activities may be those that are of little account to many people, small scale, and relatively unregulated. They may also include covert and illegal activities. More generally, informal also has a variety of meanings: It covers activities that are not defined by any identifiable set of specific rules, agreements that are not legally binding, improvised and ad hoc arrangements, and behavior that circumvents existing rules.

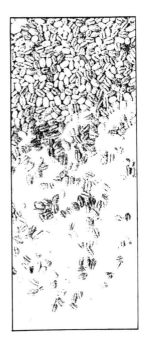

Where the Wild Things Are

Carol Laderman

In this first case study, Carol Laderman looks at the contribution children make to their individual and to household diets by foraging. The parish she studied in Malaysia stretched from the seashore to the edge of the jungle and thus contained a range of different ecological conditions and settlement patterns.

Her research demonstrates the importance of children's activities and their informal, even recreational, nature. They are often conceived of not as work but as play. Her research further shows the significance of domestic ties beyond the household. Children who join together to go foraging come from different households, and they eat cooked food at the houses of relatives, friends, and neighbors.

More generally, Laderman's analysis indicates the importance for understanding dietary practices of a detailed examination of the whole ecosystem in which people live and suggests the descriptive value of such concepts as ecological niche. In the area she studied, the extent to which households use and depend on wild greens and other products of foraging is related primarily to ecological conditions and seasonal changes, although other considerations also influence choices.

People's reliance on wild plants, particularly at certain seasons, belies their emphasis on fish and rice as the main and most necessary components of their diet. Laderman stresses that there is no simple relationship between ideology and behavior and cautions those who seek to make broad generalizations about dietary practices. The practicalities of people's lives and the particularity of their tastes can, and do in this case, lead to widespread variation.

Children's contributions to the household economy of peasant families have been evaluated primarily in terms of "adult-freeing" tasks. Detailed studies in rural South and Southeast Asia (Nag, White, and Peet 1978) have shown that, by assuming some of the duties of household maintenance and animal husbandry that would otherwise be performed by adults, children can contribute to the family's nutritional well-being by releasing their parents to perform the work that results in food, or the money to buy it. Children's direct contributions to the peasant family's diet, however, have not become a subject for serious discussion, since children under the age of fifteen, at least in those rural areas previously studied, spend a minimum of time at agricultural or income-producing tasks.

The children who lived in Merchang, the east coast village of peninsular Malaysia where I worked from 1975 to 1977, were like the Javanese and Nepalese children described by White and Peet (Nag, White, and Peet 1978) in that they performed a variety of household tasks, often from an early age. Girls of seven and eight years old were considered adequate babysitters and were also expected to help with kitchen and laundry duties. Boys could be relied on to gather firewood and could be pressed into childcare and household tasks if no suitable sister was available.

Children did not concern themselves with animal husbandry, a task that consumes a good deal of time in other peasant societies. The few goats and cattle in Merchang are allowed to wander through the parish at will. Most families keep chickens, but they require minimal care, since they eat almost every kind of garbage the housewife flings out the door or drops through the floorboards, as well as scratching for their own tidbits, and they put themselves to bed in their coops each night with no assistance from their owners.

Malay children are often clever with their hands, but unlike the Javanese children observed by White, who produced handicrafts for sale, the children of Merchang turned their skills to the fashioning of wood and metal toys, and occasionally rafts, for their own use.

Few children worked significant amounts of time on the land, with the exception of those living in a small hamlet recently carved out of the jungle, four miles from school over roads demanding goat-footed agility. Many of the less dedicated scholars in this hamlet dropped out of school to join their elders on the farm.

With the exception of those living in this pioneering community, preteenage children of this parish neither tended animals, cultivated the land, nor produced handicrafts for sale. Yet they did contribute directly to their own and their families' diets by adding wild supplements, both animal and vegetable, to the basic diet provided by their parents. Most of their foraging activities are not considered work by either the children or their elders, yet wild species collected by children and adults form a surprisingly large proportion of the diet—surprising, perhaps, because we are not in the habit of thinking of peasants as serious foragers.

THE RESEARCH SETTING

Merchang is located on the coast of the South China Sea, in the state of Trengganu, in the northeastern part of peninsular Malaysia.[1] The name Merchang is used both for the parish, comprising several villages and hamlets, and for the central village. As is the case with many coastal parishes, a large number of houses in Merchang are located close to the major highway, which roughly parallels the coastline. Unlike many other village–hamlet complexes, however, Merchang has not only been settled along the coast but extends as well approximately three miles inland to meet the jungle, which is gradually being opened for logging and agriculture. Because of its inland extension, Merchang's ecology includes seashore, river, wet rice land, primary and secondary forest, and cultivated land with both sandy and rich soils. The climate is tropical, with mean temperatures hovering around 85°F during the day, except during the monsoon season, when it drops into the 70s by day and the 60s by night. The seasons are divided into the dry season, when no rain falls for weeks on end, the monsoon (known as the cold season or the season of floods), and the months in between, when there is a moderate amount of rain.

Secondary and tertiary dirt roads lead away from the highway and into the hamlets, culminating in a mud and stick road over a swamp that connects the jungle-outpost hamlet with the rest of the world. In general, the further the hamlet is from the highway, the more dispersed is its settlement. The houses near the highway are close together, while many of those near the jungle are a quarter of a mile from their closest neighbors.

This settlement arrangement has its complementary pattern of land use. Although most families own or have access to coconut palms, people who live near the highway have no more than a few fruit trees and a tiny kitchen garden near their homes. The few who own rice land, or land planted with the cash crops of the area (rubber, tobacco, and watermelons), must travel up to three miles by bicycle or by foot to reach their plots. People who live in the inland hamlets, however, rarely have less than a half acre of fruit and coconut trees and a half-acre vegetable garden near their homes. Many inland people also have plots of land devoted to rice and cash-crop cultivation, located further from their homes but still within easy reach.

A survey of all households in four hamlets,[2] starting with one located near the highway, and continuing inland to the last, closest to the jungle, showed an obvious pattern of neolocal residence. By far, the largest percentage of people in Merchang live in a simple nuclear family (see Table 2.1). Although households (those living in the same house) that include more than two generations are relatively rare, it is common to find married children and the parents of one, or both, living in the same parish. In general, households also constitute eating units. However, adult children and their parents often bring gifts of food, both raw and cooked, to one another.

Children frequently eat meals at their grandparents' homes. They usually bring small amounts of money to school to buy snacks (usually featuring fish and rice) and may be invited for tea and cakes, or fruit, by friends and neighbors, as well as by relatives. On the way home from school, children often pick edible leaves and berries, both from plants that have been cultivated and from others growing naturally along the wayside.

T A B L E   2.1
Household Composition

Type Composition	N	Percentage
I. Single-person household	5	3.5
II. Married couple, no children	9	6.5
III. Nuclear family (married couple and children)	96	69.5
IV. Truncated nuclear (like III, but with one spouse missing because of death or divorce)	2	1.5
V. Extended vertical (three or four generations)	16	11.5
VI. Skipped-generation extended vertical	8	6.0
VII. One parent, one child, and child's spouse	1	.5
VIII. Married couple, children, and one child's spouse	1	.5
TOTAL	138	99.5

Note: Percentages may not add exactly to 100 because of rounding.

WILD FOODS IN MERCHANG

I became aware of the importance of wild foods in Merchang shortly after my arrival, since I came during the monsoon season, precisely the time when they are most needed in the diet. High waves kept the fishermen ashore, so fresh fish were unavailable. Although cultivated vegetables were nowhere to be found, I soon noticed people bringing home large bundles of greens daily. I was told that these were *daun kayu*, the generic name for wild vegetables, and that they formed a significant part of the diet, particularly during the rainy season.

In my four-hamlet survey, I collected general information regarding diet and the use of wild species. In discussions with key informants, I explored the range of wild products available and the possibilities for their use. I also collected daily dietary information covering periods of several successive days or weeks from a number of subjects. All of this information was supplemented by observations made by myself and my family. Much of the participant observation, insofar as it pertains to children's activities, was done by "remote control." My ten-year-old son, who attended the village school, accompanied his friends on their expeditions and, after being taught which wild products were edible, was able to supply our own household.

Fishing and Shellfishing

For the children of Merchang aged nine through twelve school lasts from 7 A.M. to 1 P.M. Once the school day is over, the books are put away and rarely opened until the next morning. The long daylight hours that remain offer ample opportunities for boys, and occasionally their sisters, to look for clams and snails in the mangrove swamps along the riverbanks. Feet must be bare to negotiate the mud, and one runs the risk of stepping painfully on a root protruding from the ground, but an afternoon's clamming can provide a family with enough for several meals and, sometimes, an extra basketful to sell to the neighbors. Clams are preferred to snails, but snails are eaten if nothing better presents itself. Frequently, the snails are used as excellent bait for the boys' favorite occupation, fishing.

Many boys not only fish when school is over but play hooky in order to spend more hours at this sport. Wrapping nylon line and hooks bought in village stores around pieces of wood they have found or cut for themselves, boys catch kingfish, scad, carp, catfish, climbing perch, eels, and Siamese fighting fish (for eating, and not as pets) in the swamps and paddy fields and horse mackerel, snappers, grunters, and stargazers in the river. Some children use rafts of their own making to take them down the river toward the estuary's mouth, where the fish are larger. They spend long sunny afternoons on the river, coming home before twilight (when spirit activity is at its height) by means of eddies, poling, and hand paddling. A good day's catch could obviate the necessity of their parents' spending the dollar or so it takes to buy sufficient fish for a family for that day, a significant contribution in view of the average income of M$150 a month (approximately US$65).

Wild Fruits and Vegetables

Fishing and clamming are well known throughout the world as pastimes of rural children. Foraging for wild fruits and vegetables is less expected in a peasant community, especially among people who, like the Malays, are reputed to undervalue all plant foods (Wolff 1965; Wilson 1970). Wolff reported that Malays consider fish and rice as the only foods essential to the diet. Vegetables are thought of as simply additives that improve the taste of rice, and fruits are not considered food at all, merely "pleasant things to keep the mouth busy." Malays in my parish agreed with Wolff's assessment of their food hierarchy. "Fish and rice, rice and fish, that's us," one of my neighbors remarked cheerfully.

Wilson, working just twelve miles from Merchang, found that the people of Ru Muda, a fishing village, thought of vegetables as a relish, not necessary for sustenance as are fish and rice. She concluded that there was no gardening tradition among Malay women, and that, in any case, east coast Malays are too "lazy to grow vegetables" (Wilson 1970, 140).

It would seem unlikely, under the circumstances, that Malay children or adults would spend much time either cultivating plants or gathering wild varieties, particularly in view of Firth's similar observations regarding the lack of gardens in her east coast village (1966, 93). Nevertheless, in Merchang, there is extensive cultivation of fruits and vegetables. Seventy-nine percent of all the households in my four-hamlet survey had fruit trees, and 43 percent planted vegetables, with the averages going up to 92 percent and 71 percent, respectively, in the hamlet closest to the jungle. Besides rice, seventeen varieties of vegetables and thirty-seven varieties of fruit were grown.

Merchang's complex ecology supports an even greater number of edible wild species. I counted seventy-two varieties of wild plants being eaten, some infrequently, others almost daily (see Appendix I). Consumption of wild vegetables varies considerably from hamlet to hamlet, and most variation can be explained by ecological differences. The mode for eating wild vegetables in the hamlet closest to the jungle is seven days a week; in the hamlet furthest from the jungle the mode is "never, or only during the monsoon"; and in the two intermediate hamlets the mode is one to two days a week. The range, however, is the same for all the hamlets of Merchang: Some households eat wild products every day, while others do so rarely or never (see Table 2.2). Those few households in the jungle-outpost hamlet that eat only cultivated vegetables do so because of taste preference and convenience. Those who live in the hamlet near the shore, unless they own land further inland or work on someone else's inland farm, are unlikely to gather wild vegetables frequently, since it is usually done on an opportunistic basis on the

TABLE 2.2
Wild-Vegetable Consumption in Merchang ($N = 101$)

Frequency of Consumption	Percentage of Hamlet Households				
	I	II	III	IV	Total
Monsoon only, or never	10	12	8	35	15
1 day a month			4	5	2
2 days a month	3		4		2
1 day a week	26	8	19	15	18
2 days a week	7	32	19	25	20
3 days a week	10	16	15		11
4 days a week	7	4	12		6
5 days a week	3		4	5	3
7 days a week	33	28	16	15	24
TOTAL	99	100	101	100	101

Note: This is a survey of four hamlets. I represents the hamlet closest to the jungle; II, the contiguous hamlet in the direction of the shore; III, closer to the shore; and IV, located directly on the shore. Frequency refers only to nonmonsoon months.

way home from work. They verbalize this situation by explaining that "it's too much trouble" or "I'm too lazy." Other reasons that people along the shore give for omitting wild vegetables from their diet include the presence of babies and the absence of older children in the family (which would make it difficult for the mother to go gathering), the lack of necessity for wealthier households to gather food, and, in one case, distaste for any vegetables whatsoever.

The vast majority of people in Merchang, however, know where to find and how to prepare wild foods. I was surprised by the sheer volume and variety of wild plant foods in the diet, since, in a careful study of the literature, Dunn (1975, 95) could find no reference to forest collecting by Malays, and Wilson (1970, 139) mentions their occasional use as "poverty foods" eaten only during times of necessity. Malays in Merchang do not consider wild foods fit only for emergency fare or for the tables of the poor. Neither, it would appear, do many other Malaysians. At any time of the year, at least fifteen wild varieties are sold in the markets of Kuala Trengganu, the state capital, at prices comparable to those of cultivated plants. Even in Kuala Lumpur, the nation's capital, located on the more urbanized west coast, the six or seven wild species offered for sale during most of the year command prices no lower than those of cultivated varieties.

Wild vegetables can be found everywhere in Merchang: *keladi agak*, a water plant that grows in the paddy fields; *serian*, which prefers the secondary forest; many species of fern found along the seashore; and *terung pipit*, sweet little eggplants that grow wherever the soil is rich. Palm cabbage, eaten raw or cooked with fish and coconut cream, is a welcome but infrequent addition to the diet, since it means the destruction of the tree. A particular delicacy is the *kulat sisir*, a mushroom that grows on dead rubber trees during the monsoon season.

The seeds of *buah jering, buah keredas*, and *buah petar* are gathered for local use and for sale. All are claimed to be palliatives for diabetes and, in fact, *buah jering* and *buah petar* are known to be diuretics, which could relieve the water retention common in diabetes. *Jering*, however, contains a volatile oil and an alkaloid that, if eaten in large quantities, inflames the kidneys and causes hematuria (Burkill 1966, 1792). The Malays are aware of this danger. To prevent it, they boil *jering* in two or three changes of water and keep them for a day before eating.

Young shoots and leaves, sometimes of large trees, are plucked at all times of the year. Adults gather armfuls of wild greens on their way back from work. Children may pick some for their own enjoyment when walking back from school or playing, but they must be specifically asked to pick enough salad for the family's supper—not because it is an onerous task, since the ingredients can easily be found close to home, but because it seems more like work, while fishing seems like play.

Children never have to be coaxed to gather wild fruits. They are their principal consumers. Most wild fruits have a short season, so with the passing of the months the children's taste treats change. In February and March they hit wild mangosteens off the trees with long poles; from April through August they do the same to the sweet little red fruits of *kayu kelat*. From January through May, children climb the *gucil* tree to pick its fruit; in July and August, it is the *sisek puyu*'s turn. Fruits that grow on bushes are easier to pick casually as the children pass by: the tiny tart red *buah binan setukar*, the sweet little white *buah gelam tikus*, the black *buah terajang*, yellow *buah ulat bulu*, and the *buah keduduk*, whose sweet blue fruits were once used for ink as well as for eating.

Some fruits, such as *buah kemunting*, gathered by children the year round, attract adults as well during their peak season (October through December), when there is enough to satisfy everyone's appetite and still leave an abundance to sell to city people. Children rarely venture into the jungle alone, but during October and November large parties of children and adults spend whole days there collecting wild fruits, such as *buah kelubi, buah salak*, and *buah rekan*, and wild chestnuts (*buah berangan* and *geratak tangga*), which are fried in a pan along with clean sand, then peeled and eaten as a snack or pounded and made into cakes.

Children's contributions to the family diet increase in importance during the monsoon season, when most paying work is at a standstill and incomes are at their lowest. Cultivated vegetables are unavailable, and, because of hazardous fishing conditions, fresh fish are nowhere to be found. Wild vegetables are particularly relished at this time, and many households whose usual consumption occurs about four times a week increase their use of wild plants to at least once a day.

School, too, is closed during the monsoon. The shellfish gathered by children provide a welcome change in a monsoon diet that otherwise relies heavily on dried salted fish for its animal protein. In this time of enforced vacation from other chores, both children and adults have the leisure to collect and prepare wild products that are not normally eaten because they are toxic unless prepared by a lengthy process: *paku piah*, a fern that must be boiled in at least three changes of water; *jeneris*, a climber, which is boiled twice and kept for two days before eating; and *buah berus*, the fruit of a tall tree, which must have its outer skin scraped thoroughly before it is boiled in three changes of water. Use of these toxic plants depends upon the relative availability of other, preferred, foods. The first monsoon season I spent in Merchang, large quantities of *buah berus* supplemented the dried fish and rice diet. During the second monsoon season, there were shipments of fresh fish from the west coast (which experiences its own rainy season during other months of the year), and consumption of *buah berus* went down considerably.

SIGNIFICANCE OF WILD FOODS IN THE DIET

If the profusion of fruits and vegetables eaten in Merchang appears to conflict with Malay dietary conceptions, the quantities consumed present an even more striking example of the differences between ideology and behavior. It is true that Malays think of vegetables as a relish, not absolutely essential for survival or strength. Nutritional status, however, does not depend upon ideas stated by one's lips but on the food that passes between them. Portions of vegetables consumed in Merchang are considerably larger than one might expect from a food in the relish category: 40 to 230 grams per meal, as compared to a typical American serving of 70 to 80 grams per meal (U.S. Department of Agriculture 1978). Sixty-four percent of all households in my four-hamlet survey ate a serving of green or yellow vegetables at least once a day, and 35 percent usually had vegetables twice a day (Laderman 1983, 30). Wild vegetables represent almost half of all vegetable products eaten in Merchang. While nutritive values for most edible wild plants have not yet been computed, such common varieties as *cekor manis*, a green leafy vegetable, have been shown to contribute significant amounts of vitamins A and C to the diet, comparing favorably with cultivated species.

Wild plants assume further importance in the postpartum period. According to the Malay theory of humors, a woman who has recently given birth and therefore lost blood, the "hot" body humor, is in a "cold" state for forty days thereafter. During this time, it is believed wise to eat foods considered humorally "hot" or neutral and to avoid humorally "cold" foods. Many cultivated vegetables are considered "cold," but several wild plants are "hot." Others, if eaten separately, are neutral, but if mixed together as a raw salad they are thought to become "hot." (See Laderman 1979, 66, and Laderman 1983, 39, for specific information on these varieties.) The use of wild plants in the Malay traditional postpartum diet can contribute needed nutrients during this time of physiological stress. The presence of a child who may be relied on to gather wild plants can be important to women following a postpartum restricted diet whose husbands are temporarily working far from home (a fairly common occurrence), as well as to those in the last stages of pregnancy, or with a nursing infant, whose diets are not restricted but whose movements may be.

The picture I have painted of the bewildering variety of edible plants eaten in Merchang contrasts vividly with Wilson's description of the Malay diet. The people of Merchang and the people of Ru Muda (Wilson's research site) share the same religion, social organization, history, and traditions. They would both be characterized as peasants in any standard anthropology textbook. Yet we appear to be discussing two populations separated by years of history or miles of terrain, rather than two groups of east coast Malays living only twelve miles apart.

Their dietary differences can be understood only in the light of ecological and demographic differences. Their differential use of plants cannot be explained by differences in education, socio-economic status, or changing values stemming from modernization or culture contact. The significant variables are the availability of plants, the ecology that supports them, and the subsistence activities related to exploitation of the ecology.

Ru Muda is a seaside fishing community built on sandy soil that is not conducive to agriculture. Although it is possible to cultivate the soil, conditions in this ecological zone make gardening unprofitable. Fishing, however, is a very profitable activity in Ru Muda. Its proximity to coral reefs and offshore islands makes it a center for fishing and fish drying. One can always tell when one has reached Ru Muda by the overpowering odor of drying fish. The time and effort that go into catching and drying fish, which might otherwise be spent in inland gardening, bring good returns to the people.

Because of the importance of their fishing industry, the inhabitants of Ru Muda have settled near the beaches and have not penetrated deeply inland.[3] One would expect to find few wild fruits and vegetables thriving within easy reach, and that, in fact, is the case. In Merchang, with the exception of large parties that form for the exploitation of jungle resources in season, wild fruits and vegetables are usually collected opportunistically every day. Were one to assume that a similar pattern would prevail in Ru Muda, one would not expect wild plants to form any significant part of the diet, a hypothesis borne out by Wilson's observations (1970, 139). The differences between Ru Muda's ecology and diet and those of Merchang point up the need for microecological studies and provide a caveat to those who too easily make generalizations, whether ecological, dietary, or related to any other sphere of human existence and behavior.[4]

In spite of their food ideology, which favors rice and fish and devalues fruits and vegetables, rural Malays, in practice, appear to prefer the varied diet possible only in settlements located in an ecological zone that supports such variety or in villages within easy reach of a market. Children who live in a rich ecological zone like Merchang, because of their foraging and gathering activities, can be seen as contributors to, rather than merely consumers of, the domestic economy.

POSTSCRIPT

As I began to think about writing this chapter, a transformation occurred, so gradually and stealthily that I scarcely knew it was happening. What had started out to be a lighthearted account of Huck Finn on the banks of the South China Sea had inexorably broadened into a discussion of the significance of foraging in peasant societies and the importance of ecological particularization. The logic of this transformation lies at the heart of the anthropological vision. For just as a joke or a slip of the tongue may carry messages to a psychologist about the workings of the human mind, an investigation of children's pastimes by an anthropologist must inevitably lead to consideration of larger issues concerning the human condition.

APPENDIX I: Edible Wild Plants
Consumed in Merchang

Vegetables

1. Balek adab (Fam. Rubiaceae, possibly *Mussaenda* sp.)
2. Bayam ngang (Fam. Compositae)
3. Bayam peraksi (Fam. Compositae)
4. Binan setukar (*Decaspermum frutenscens* Fam. Myrtaceae)
5. Cekor manis (*Sauropus androgynus*)
6. Deber lembu (Fam. Compositae)
7. Gajah nangis (*Saraca* sp. Fam. Leguminosae)
8. Gelam tikus (*Eugenia* sp.)
9. Gucil (*Antidesma ghaesembillau* Fam. Euphorbiaceae)
10. Jeneris (*Connarus ellipticus*)
11. Kayu kelat (*Eugenia* sp. Mytacaea)
12. Keladi agak (*Monochoria vaginalis* Fam. Pontederiacerae)
13. Kerkoh batu (*Myrica esculenta* Fam. Myricaceae)
14. Kulat batu (*Lentinus sajor-caju*)
15. Kulat sisir (*Schizophyllum*)
16. Kulat telinga tikus (*Auricularia auriculae-judae*)
17. Lapeng budak (*Clerodendron* sp. Fam. Verbenaceae)

18. Leban (*Vitex pubescens* Fam. Verbenaceae)
19. Lidah katung (unidentified)
20. Paku hijau (*Ceropteris*)
21. Paku merah (*Nephrodium*)
22. Paku piah (*Cycus* cfr. *rumphii* Fam. Cycadaceae)
23. Pinan keroh (*Cnestis palala* Fam. Connaraceae)
24. Pokok kuat (*Ploiarium alterniforium Melch.* Fam. Myricaceae)
25. Pucuk midin (*Stenochlaena palustris*)
26. Putak (*Barringtonia* sp. Fam. Lecythidacedae)
27. Rebung buluh (*Bambusa*: bamboo shoots)
28. Sawa hubu (possibly Fam. Thizophoraceae or Fam. Rubiaceae)
29. Sepit (either *Sesuvium portulacastrium* or *Portulaca oleraceae*)
30. Serai kayu (unidentified)
31. Serian (*Cissus* sp. Fam. Vitaceae)
32. Sisek puyu (*Carallia*)
33. Sugidama (possibly *Guioa* Fam. Sapindaceae)
34. Terung pipit (*Solanum torvum*)
35. Tudung periok (Fam. Rubiaceae, probably an *Ixora* sp.)
36. Ulat bulu (*Passiflora foetida*)

Edible Palm Cabbages, Obtained from Wild and Domesticated Individuals of the Following Species:

1. Umbuk bayas (*Oncosperma horrida*)
2. Umbuk kelapa (*Cocos*)
3. Umbuk nibung (*Oncosperma tigillaria*)
4. Umbuk palas (*Licuala*)
5. Umbuk pinang (*Areca*)

Fruits

1. Asam gelugor (*Garcinia* sp.)
2. Buah berangan (*Castanopsis* sp. Fam. Fagaceae)
3. Buah beruas (*Garnicia hombroniana* Fam. Guttiferae)
4. Buah berus (*Bruguiera parviflora*)
5. Buah binan setukar (*Descaspermun frutenscens* Fam. Myrtaceae)
6. Buah gelam tikus (*Eugenia zeylanica*)
7. Buah gucil (*Antidesma ghaesembilla* Fam. Euphorbiaceae)
8. Buah jentik (*Baccaurea*)

9. Buah jering (*Pithecellobium jiringa*)
10. Buah kandis (*Garcinia* sp.)
11. Buah kayu kelat (*Eugenia* sp. Mytacaea)
12. Buah keduduk (*Melastoma malabathricum*)
13. Buah kelubi (*Zalacca* sp.)
14. Buah kemunting (*Rhodomyrtus tomentosa*)
15. Buah keredas (*Pithecellobium microcarpus*)
16. Buah kerkoh batu (*Myrica esculenta* Fam. Myricaceae)
17. Buah mata ayam (*Ardisia crispa*)
18. Buah mata kucing (*Nephelium malaiense*)
19. Buah nipah (*Nipa fruticans*)
20. Buah palas (*Licuala* sp. Fam. Palmae)
21. Buah petar (*Parkia speciosa*)
22. Buah rekan (*Zalacca* sp.)
23. Buah salak (*Zalacca* sp.)
24. Buah setial (*Sendoricum* sp.)
25. Buah setol (*Sendoricum indicum*)
26. Buah sisik puyu (*Carallia*)
27. Buah terajang (*Erioglossum rubiginosum*)
28. Buah ulat bulu (*Passiflora foetida*)
29. Geratak tangga (*Castanopsis* sp. Fam. Fagaceae)
30. Nyior lemba (*Curculigo* sp. Fam. Hypoxidaceae)
31. Rambutan gerat, also known as buah pahit (*Nephelium mutabile*)

Note: These plants were identified by Professor Benjamin C. Stone formerly of the Department of Botany, University of Malaya. The division into fruits and vegetables was done by my informants in Merchang. *Buah* usually refers to fruit, *umbuk* to palm cabbage, *paku* to fern, and *kulat* to fungi.

NOTES

Acknowledgments: Research on which this chapter is based was supported by the Social Science Research Council, the Danforth Foundation, National Institute of Mental Health Training Grant 5 F31 MHO5 352-03, and by the University of California International Center for Medical Research through research grant AI 10051 to the Department of Epidemiology and International Health, University of California, San Francisco, from the National Institute of Allergy and Infectious Diseases, National Institutes of Health, U.S. Public Health Services. It was done under the auspices of the Institute for Medical Research of the Malaysian Ministry of Health.

1. My description of Merchang refers to conditions during 1975, 1976, and 1977. When I returned in 1982 I noticed that several major changes had occurred; for example, a real road had been built linking the jungle-outpost hamlet with the rest of the parish. Use of wild foods continues as described in this chapter.

2. The four hamlets in which I conducted intensive surveys represent about one-third of the population of Merchang. These contiguous hamlets encompassed all the ecological and demographic conditions in the area: Their locations ranged from seashores to newly cleared jungle; their houses were located at various distances from each other, ranging from about twenty feet in the seaside hamlet to almost a quarter of a mile in the jungle outpost; their land use varied from small kitchen gardens near the home and plots of land further away to sizeable farms close to home; and their residents' place of origin varied from mostly natives of Merchang and environs in the seaside hamlet to an entirely immigrant population (from Kelantan) in the jungle outpost.

3. The Firths also chose a fishing village as their research site since the focus of Raymond Firth's study was the Malay fishermen's economy. He noted that the fisherfolk had "elaborate and intimate social relations with the agricultural sector of the population" (1966, 5); however, his wife (Rosemary Firth 1966, 93) observed that there did "not seem to be any tradition that a fisherman's wife would do gardening on any scale," an observation wholly in accord with Wilson's and my own in relation to Ru Muda.

4. I have recently learned, with great interest, that patterns of wild plant use comparable to those in Merchang are to be found in other parts of Malaysia with similar ecological conditions (Massard 1983, 172–76).

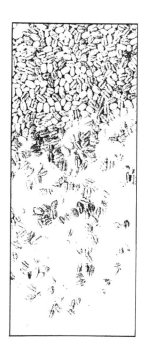

CHAPTER 3

Getting Through (Three) Meals a Day: Diet, Domesticity, and Cash Income in a Mexican Community

Ellen Messer

Using an eclectic approach, Ellen Messer addresses questions about the interrelations between women's activities and allocation of time, their income production and use, and the diet and health of themselves and the members of their domestic units. Some of the questions addressed were raised by such early writers as Richards (1939) and have continued to concern researchers in anthropology, nutrition, economics, and various policy areas for many years without any very satisfactory answers being produced.

Messer's particular contribution in this chapter is to present a method she has developed for intensive observation and analysis of what household members actually do: their interactions with, and care of, young children; how they spend their days; how they obtain and use money; and how and where they eat and distribute food. Few writers have collected information on these topics by direct observation or developed a method that enables them to trace the working out of the interrelations between different aspects of people's lives over time.

Her analysis demonstrates the variability in time use and activities among households and within the same household from day to day. As she follows women and children she shows how households (though residential, culinary, budgeting, and commensal units) merge into larger residential or social groupings of which they are a part. Her observations, like Laderman's, indicate that all household members, even young children, are active in trying to provide for their own needs. Finally, she suggests why there can be no single, standard answer to the question of why certain households thrive and others fail nutritionally under the "same" cultural, economic, and nutritional conditions.

T he complex linkages between nutrient intake and social performance receive attention from both anthropologists and nutritionists. Especially, the interconnections between the activity profiles of focal women, the social organization of households, and the abilities of individual women to organize household resources are important in determining individual nutrient intakes within households. Household heads must manage effectively both material resources and the other household personnel in order to provide adequate nutrients and other forms of care to household members, particularly children.

Various ethnographic and nutritional studies suggest that the nutritional status of the focal woman of the household affects her ability to organize and care for the household (Messer 1984a, 432–33, 444–5, 455–60; 1984b, 235–36). Any deterioration in her household maintenance in turn affects the work performance and health of herself and the other members of the household. Reciprocally, her income and that of other household members, in the context of the particular household organization, influence how well she functions and provides food.

The object of this study, carried out in Mitla, Oaxaca, Mexico, was to determine how focal women's activity patterns, especially cash-remunerated work (a measure of social performance) affects household organization, food choices, nutrient intake, and health. Although the data and occupational structure are specific to this town, the observations on household time and food management are applicable more generally to contexts inside and outside Mexico, both in cases where businessmen enter villages to organize women's domestic production (embroidering, crocheting, sewing) for nonlocal markets and also in urban areas, where women assume responsibility for some or most of household income through food processing and other service occupations.

Direct observations of focal women's time allocations were used to determine how the exigencies of household maintenance tasks—including food preparation, child feeding, general health care, and hygiene—affected productive work for cash. Conversely, the method also showed how cash work interfered with household duties. Specific questions included: (1) whether women spent more or less time in food acquisition, preparation, feeding, and cleanup under different occupational regimes; (2) how the household organization of tasks was adjusted to allow them to complete cash-earning tasks, or how household responsibilities limited their ability to earn income; (3) what accommodations were made in dietary planning and household maintenance (for example, sanitation tasks and laundry) where cash work competed with time needed for food provisioning, household maintenance, and child care; (4) if there were easily calculable nutritional differences, based on food intake, among households with different occupational structures that made different demands on women's time for cash work.

ETHNOGRAPHIC BACKGROUND AND METHODS

The Mitla, Oaxaca, study was part of a ten-year perspective on the town. Observations from the first nine years were incorporated in the selection of households[1] for time use observations during the tenth year. Over the first part of the tenth year, background data on women's productive and reproductive histories in the context of their household economies were collected in 150 households as part of a more general study of changing household economies over this period. I visited, participant-observed, and informally interviewed both men and women in households to assess the direct and indirect impact of government socioeconomic policies on their changing activity patterns. I recorded household histories, the ages and numbers of children, the material standard of living, the usual eating and working patterns, and any particular health problems.

In the second part of the study, 20 of these 150 households were selected for more intensive day-long studies of activity and dietary patterns.[2] Each household was observed on four days—two during the rainy season and two during the dry season, which corresponded to the "vacation" and school seasons, respectively—to capture variability in both natural and cultural seasonal activities and eating patterns. Each observation day began at 7 A.M. when the author or a trained research assistant (Yale B.A. in political science, female) entered the household to keep a time record of all activities of the focal woman and of all children and other adults around her. As the day progressed, the observer noted starting and stopping times of all activities (and social interactions), including conversations and other behaviors, by a simple diary method. She afterward summed the duration of all episodes of each activity in standardized activity types—food preparation, household maintenance, child care, leisure (which included rest, personal hygiene, and eating), cash work, visiting, food acquisition (which included shopping and foraging)—and then calculated the total time allotted to each activity type over the day.[3]

Profiles of individual women's activity patterns—in time and percentage of time over the twelve-hour period of observation (7 A.M. to 7 P.M.)—were calculated and compared to show the ranges and dimensions of variation of activity patterns and diets within the "same" culture or even the same person. Observations also revealed how cash work significantly interfered with or dominated decisions regarding food. In addition, individual household accounts provided complete records of how children acquire food in situations where they are *not* being fed well by parents (in either the parents' or the observer's view).

The timed activity data were complemented by data on household dietary intakes and expenditures. To measure how women's activities affected food intake, individual nutrient intakes were recorded. The daily rhythm of household life was disturbed only during eating occasions, when the recorder weighed and calculated costs of ingredients that went into meal preparation and measured and weighed all food portions ingested by each household member. Snacks consumed by children and other household members during the day also were recorded. This involved following children around while the focal woman was occupied with a repetitive task, such as food preparation or sewing. Children were also questioned about what they had eaten after they returned home. (Adults reported what they had eaten outside the household as they returned.) Casual observations of household meal and snacking patterns on nonstudy days provided insights into snacking behaviors and also into the representativeness of the study day observations.

To understand how women's activities affected cash income and purchases, household expenditures were recorded. Expenses included outlays for food (also, where relevant, calculations of consumption in kind, as where a household might have its own maize supply), plus daily or weekly outlays for personal and laundry soap; flowers and candles for the saints; and time payments on dishes, pans, beds, sewing machines, and other articles (trade patterns were noted also). Exceptional expenditures, disrupting meal schedules and ordinary budget outlays, were observed in two cases; contributions to funeral feasts preempted household needs in both instances.

THE TOWN AND THE SAMPLE

Mitla is a town of approximately nine thousand people, almost all of whom are involved to some degree in producing and marketing tourist textiles and other small items. While in 1971 approximately half of Mitla households still farmed (maize, beans, and squash), by 1981 most households were buying the better part of their food at the central marketplace or at smaller foodshops in their neighborhoods: They had turned to occupations that were more reliable and remunerative than agriculture. Although they might still farm a small piece of land, and keep such houseyard animals as poultry and pigs for home consumption or for sale, most comestibles, even maize, were purchased.

Maize tortillas are the staple of the diet, although many women now purchase them from professional tortilla makers rather than preparing them at home. The usual meal pattern includes a hot beverage with sweet rolls in the early morning, followed by a midmorning "meal" (*almuerzo*) of tortillas, a main dish (such as beans or pasta), and a picant sauce; a main afternoon "meal" (*comida*), also based on tortillas and a main dish and sauce; and finally an evening "coffee" that duplicates the morning repast. Between meals, people—especially children—snack on fruits, sweets, and sweet beverages. The daily cost of feeding a family of two adults and three young children in 1981 ranged from a bare minimum of

50 pesos (a peso in 1981 was worth about $.04 U.S.), for a diet that would not include meat, milk, or many condiments, to 90 pesos (the average range), or more. Families with four or more children usually spend more than 100 pesos per day on food. Most households followed a weekly cycle of beans, rice, and pasta, with meat on Sundays (and more often if they could afford it).

During the same period, the average daily wage for men was 110 to 150 pesos. Craftsmen, paid by the piece, earned a higher or lower figure depending on the numbers of garments they were able to turn out in a day. Agricultural laborers earned closer to the minimum (plus meals) except during the height of the harvest, when short supply forced wages up to between 130 and 140 pesos.

Against this background, both women and children supplemented household income by food processing, small crafts, and trade. A woman who ground one and a half kilos of maize into tortillas for regular customers could count on 15 pesos for the morning's efforts. Diligent crocheting of "flowers" that could then be latched into blouses might also net 15 pesos. Sewing (piecework) at 3–5 pesos a garment might yield 60–100 pesos, but producing twenty garments or more was considered to be extremely taxing, and many women mentioned it was "bad for the lungs" to continue at this rate. The merchant's trade, if one was an accomplished salesperson, was considerably more lucrative. Although merchants were reluctant to tell what they had paid for items, on good days they could return from the local artisans' market with 1,000 pesos or more.

All of these trades, their hours, and their responsibilities were considered in designing the household sample for intensive observations of how women managed time (see Table 3.1). Women in all twenty sample households worked, although two had begun to work only recently because they found their husbands' incomes insufficient to keep the family in food. With two exceptions, all had young children. In both of these "childless" households, women spent more than an hour every day caring for young children, including providing them with snacks, so they contributed to the total analysis of the networks by which children receive food and other kinds of care.

Since the research emphasized how women manage time, we observed two households without male providers. One was that of a spinster; the other, that of a three-generation female extended family. Neither of these is a usual household form in Mitla, from the local or the observer's point of view. Most households rely on a male spouse or older male children for at least some of their income, even where the focal woman earns the more regular and significant share of the household income.

In the sample, seven women make tortillas, twelve sew, two make dolls, two tie macrame shawls, seven crochet, and two process food. All but one household and most focal women practice multiple cash-earning activities. In addition, two women are traders. At least 300 women in Mitla trade in tourist items, either in the town or in regional markets; with difficulty, we followed the arrangements two women made around their work for child care and food provision. It was difficult to follow the women and their children in ordinary times; during the year of observation, there was the additional complication that women were trying to organize unions and syndicates to protect their selling rights in the vicinity of the Mitla Ruins. As a result, they were perhaps even busier than usual, and all outside observers were suspected (by their colleagues, not by the women themselves) of trying to get information for their adversaries.

In addition, for a woman to swap roles with her spouse and earn the main income while he or someone else provides principal child care for their offspring is not the accepted pattern for women's roles in Mitla. Our presence provided another element in the continual pressure on these women traders, principally by their mothers-in-law, to stay at home rather than pursue trade. This was true especially during the limited season of observation, since the mothers-in-law used the observers as an audience to vent their frustration at the life-styles of their sons' families. We therefore spent days with them at home as well as in the marketplace, according to their schedules and their desires to placate their spouses and in-laws. We also made a point of spending time discussing the project with their spouses and spouses' families to make sure that our presence was not complicating the young women's already difficult situation.

SUMMARY OF RESULTS

Food Intake in Relation to Household Structure

The most striking difference in dietary quantity and quality was be-tween the poorest and all other households. The two poorest households (#1 and #6, judged by daily income and material stan-dard of living) ate fewer daily meals, less food in general, and prac-ticed more foraging at all age levels than the others. In household #1, the father was out of work; the mother took in sewing when it was available. Otherwise, she made tortillas in the morning for sale or crocheted or did both. On two of the four observation days, the family ate only one main meal. The children whined continually for food and raided the mother's foodbasket when she returned from the marketplace. In this household, more evidently than in any other, food was withheld as punishment if children did not perform their household chores or otherwise displeased the mother. She, in turn, was irritable and lacked stamina in performing her chores. She, with relatives and neighbors, also foraged regularly for fire fuel, which saved them the expense of purchasing wood. When there was no sewing to earn cash, the opportunity cost of foraging was low and the diversionary value was high. During the rainy sea-son, such trips were combined with foraging for edible mushrooms and edible wild greens; later, at harvest time, with gleaning (maize and beans). When there was no cash in the house, they bought goods on credit from one or another store or borrowed from a near relative or *compadre* (godparent of one of the children). The oldest boy, fourteen, and the oldest girl, eleven, worked with the husband and wife, respectively, on their tasks and so contributed to household maintenance and income.

In this household, the mother "got through the day" with the help of her oldest daughter, who did most of the household chores. After they both arose before 6 A.M. to wash the maize boiled the night before with lime, the girl went to the mill to grind maize for tortillas at six o'clock, then helped with food preparation (the morning coffee) and cleanup, cared for the infant, and washed the laundry, while the mother ground and marketed tortillas. When she returned from selling tortillas, the mother would bring with her some food to prepare the one main family meal. Then she would do additional household chores, more laundry (which was never ending, given the infant), and begin her income-producing activities. If there was no sewing, she crocheted, which yielded a low return for time expended, but at least a certain return (10–15 pesos, which would purchase one to two kilos of maize for three or four hours' labor)—a pittance to get by on. If there was sewing, she often worked far into the night to finish an order. She was exhausted most of the time, and as we learned later she was also pregnant with their sixth child, although she was still occasionally giving the breast to the youngest child, already two years old and eating other liquid and solid adult foods, but *not* milk or any high nutrient quality products, which were too expensive for the family's household budget.

In similar fashion, a related household (#6) in the neighborhood got through the day with two sparse meals of tortillas and chili sauce, and sometimes a bit of egg or greens. The two focal women (mother and daughter), with the help of the twelve-year-old granddaughter, ground tortillas in the early mornings. Then the daughter went to sell them and returned around midday with whatever groceries and sundries they would need that day. She would then set to work crocheting, earning 10–15 pesos in the afternoon, while the mother either crocheted or tied the ends of macrame shawls. If there was a shortage of piecework (shawls), the mother, with the aid of the daughter or granddaughter, would also take in washing from wealthier households. This wash was done at her well or taken to the nearby river. Washing yielded a good return (20 pesos per dozen pieces, perhaps 40 pesos for a heavy afternoon's work) for the time allocated (although the labor was more taxing physically than either of the crafts) and also supplied soap, the excess of which could be used to launder their own clothes.

Mother and daughter also took in maize to make tortillas on consignment for festivals. They received a set fee to produce a fixed number of tortillas per kilo of maize (15 pesos per *almud*—volume weighs between 3 and 4 kilos—30 pesos for a hard morning's work), plus the leftover maize for their own consumption (usually enough for their daily intake). Their earnings, in every case, went directly into food and other daily expenditures. The 12-year-old helped them in all of these tasks and, in addition, contributed substantially to caring for her visiting half-sisters. If there was no money to purchase maize for the next day's food processing (as was the case when they laid out money for funeral expenses), one or more of the women would crochet to earn enough (15 pesos) to purchase maize to begin operations again. As was the case in household #1, the women (often all three generations) met in the late afternoon to forage for food and for fuel, which saved them the additional expense of purchasing firewood. When they had no cash to buy food, they, too, would try to purchase goods on credit at one or another store, would borrow from a near relative or *compadre*, or would barter tortillas for such comestibles as eggs and beans. While all of the children had learned to snatch food from the family holdings when they could, the middle son of household #1, who was generally disobedient and continually being denied food as punishment, had also become a successful forager. He picked wild fruits in the fields, nibbled at others' houses, and, during the school season, begged snacks from a godparent.

Other households were in less desperate straits. They regularly ate two meals a day, with at least another "coffee" in the morning and often in the evening as well. Furthermore, their food purchases were 50–100 percent above the minimum they could spend and still provide a sparse, though for adults adequate, diet. The women worked and in certain cases, as in household #11, specifically entered the labor force to earn money to spend on milk, fruits, and other items that they could not regularly afford on their husbands' earnings. In household #11, where the mother regularly made an extra 15–30 pesos worth of tortillas (minus 8 pesos for maize and firewood) for sale each morning, she said it was to "pay for the food" they wanted to feed their family. Her husband, although he was regularly employed as a mason, did not earn enough to cover daily outlays for extras—like milk for their infant—over and above their other purchases. Where mothers did not take this additional initiative, babies drank adult "coffee" (coffee-flavored sugar water) in nursing bottles or from cups, gummed tortilla strips prepared especially for them, and ate bits of *sopas* (tortillas moistened in gravy from beans or other dishes) for protein. Up to 40 percent of the energy intake of two- to three-year-olds might be sugar (Messer 1986).

Despite women's economic contribution, in only one household (#19) did the two main meals of the day regularly include animal protein. In this household, snacks for the children consisted of milk and other high nutrient quality foods. Coffee was replaced by milk or chocolate, and the breads, instead of being cheaper varieties made from flour and sugar, were always egg-based, expensive pieces. This household was not "rich," but the mother, who sewed pants for an international-tourist market, had decided to spend her earnings on food for her children. Her husband's income, meanwhile, went to meet the other household expenses. The mother spent most of her time cooking, feeding, and cleaning up after her two young children; she then would sew far into the night to complete a clothing order.

Most households fell somewhere in between the poorest (one meal daily) and the best fed (two meals a day with animal protein) just described. Households #4 and 5, for example, were both "tortilla" households. Like #1 and #6 focal women had the benefit of adolescent daughters' labor to help them earn cash and perform household chores. The mother in household #4 supplemented her income by macrame or crocheting; the mother in household #5 sewed and crocheted. Either of these households was better off than households #1 and 6, in that they regularly ate two meals a day. In addition, household #5 had a petroleum stove and household #4 a gas stove, each of which relieved the drudgery (or alternatively, the expense) of firewood acquisition.

Households #10 and 20 were both merchant households, in which the women did the food marketing and prepared the morning coffee, and usually the *almuerzo* and *comida*, before they left in the morning to sell. They had "house husbands" who, while carrying on crafts production (weaving, dollmaking), also took care of the children. In each case, their households had gas stoves, and the husbands could simply heat up the meal the mother had left. Alternatively, if the husband was away (since in both cases the husbands were also long-distance traders who took week-long trips), the children were left with a grandmother, usually the mother's mother, who fed and cared for them while the mother was gone during the day. Mothers would do household chores, especially the never-ending laundry, in the evenings after returning from work, early in the mornings before leaving for work, or on the one day a week they usually took off; their choice depended on the number of tourists, their supplies of goods on hand, and the exigencies of the chores. After they were weaned, children only occasionally accompanied parents to the artisan markets. When they did, they wandered around different stalls, where they were often fed snacks by the other Mitla tradeswomen, who were very often their relatives or godparents.

Finally, one should mention household #7, in which the mother began sewing, crocheting, and trading during the research period. She was trying to ensure an income for food and other household purchases as her husband sank into alcoholism. She fitted in sewing and crocheting with little enthusiasm, since she preferred to spend her time cooking, cleaning, and playing with her four children. On Sundays, she took the whole brood with her to the regional market, where she and other relatives sold clothing to tourists. The main Sunday meal was cooked the night before and reheated over a charcoal brazier they borrowed from another Mitla vendor. To make ends meet, she borrowed from her mother-in-law; this grandmother, in turn, had a claim on her granddaughters' services for various household tasks and errands. The mother, who was pregnant with her fifth child, appeared to be exhausted.

ALLOCATING TIME: DO THE MEALS SUFFER?

Unless they were nursing, women fitted in meals and other household chores around their work, rather than vice versa. Some operated efficiently on a schedule, eating regular meals at regular hours. Mealtimes were almost always dictated by the husband's work schedule, her own selling schedule, or the demands of putting out piecework. To guarantee some income, women plodded through a certain number of garments to complete an order of piecework before they would take a break to fix a meal. Children adapted to such irregular eating schedules by snacking at home or at school or by foraging. Very young children constantly whined for food, but by age four or five both boys and girls had learned to snack before meals by raiding household cupboards for bread or crackers or by making small tacos and sandwiches, usually with the permission of the mother. The parents usually had on hand such junk foods as doughnuts and crackers, in addition to coffee-flavored sugar water, to keep the children happy while they, the parents, continued to work.

Such snacking behaviors were particularly striking in children recovering from illness. Food diaries showed that they ate almost continually—whatever was on hand, in a phenomenon we termed "catch up eating"—as they were similarly noted to underconsume during active episodes of fevers and respiratory ills. Children also foraged, in that they were usually fed if they wandered into a grand-mother's or aunt's house in an extended family compound (the usual form of residence). Interfering most with mothers' work schedules were very young children who were hungry every few hours and often sick. Infants were suckled on demand, an activity interfering noticeably with mothers' economic pursuits. Younger children needing constant attention were handled by delegating child care, if possible, to a sibling aged five years or older. If none were available, the desperate mother either brought her very young child(ren) to another house for safekeeping or invited another child into the compound to amuse her own while she carried on pressing economic activities.

Choices of meal components were dictated by both budget and time. On high work load days, the meal was usually either beans (which on a gas stove or petroleum burner did not have to be watched) or a quick tomato sauce, with eggs, cheese, pork crack-lings, or sausages. When there was more time, there was some attempt, within financial constraints, at variety. The usual round during any given week for any family except the poorest was a cycle of beans, pasta, rice, eggs with salsa, and, in all but the poorest households, meat at least once a week, on Sunday if possible. Meat consumption was limited by time, as well as by income, since meat generally took not only more income but more time to prepare. However, small tidbits of meat in lieu of eggs or cheese were often consumed as garnishes to the starchy staple dishes.

Meals and snack foods improved when women worked, as a result of the extra income that could be targeted to go directly into the daily food budget. Where men provided minimal or no funds, women's income went directly into the budget for food and other necessities. In households where women earned sufficient income from food processing (as in household #2, where the women processed maize and cacao into daily income from tortillas and weekly or biweekly income from chocolate), the focal woman was responsible for the food budget, her husband for other expenditures. This pattern of separation of male and female income and budgets was noted also in other households. In each case, the men were or had been long-distance traders; therefore, it is possible that this division of labor, income, and budgets began during a period when women were unable to count on any daily or weekly income from men and had learned to fend for themselves. Food processing or very small scale trade (often in low cost items like food) was the least capital intensive manner in which to establish a regular, if marginal, income.

An additional aspect of the women's employment situation was the "trickle down" effect. Women who spent most of their time producing goods for the market, or selling there, employed other women to make tortillas, prepare daily meals, and do laundry. Thus, women's employment in manufacturing and trade had the potential to improve the diets of both their own households and those of poorer women, who earned income serving them. Alternatively, women press children into service. Girls begin to perform household tasks, especially child care and errands, by age five; these save the mother steps, particularly during food preparation. Within a few years, girls are cooking, carrying, washing clothes, and otherwise losing their playtimes to real world work. Even boys may be asked to do "women's work," including carrying maize to the mill, sweeping, making coffee and eggs, and washing out clothes if there is not enough female labor of the right age to perform such tasks, especially if the mother is working for cash in addition (households #13 and #14). The households where the meals were most irregular were those where the mothers were sewing and had not trained or disciplined their children to help regularly with the household chores. Girls were observed (impressionistically) to be more tractable than boys; boys were obedient only to the extent that they had fathers who enforced discipline. Women varied considerably in their skills and effectiveness in organizing household activities and child labor.

INTRAHOUSEHOLD FOOD DISTRIBUTION

The ordinary pattern of food distribution within the household is senior man first; oldest to youngest children according to sex, boys first; and the food preparer, usually the mother, last. Where little girls took over the mother's food serving chores, they followed this pattern scrupulously, serving their fathers first, then siblings in chronological order, then themselves. Even though they are served last, there is a general rule across households that the youngest child is favored with relatively more food, as well as other signs of affection, over other children. The child still at the breast, or the youngest child, receives the choicest morsels of protein or fruits in mealtimes and snacks over the other children. They are also favored with immediate gratification should food be available and should they demand it during the day. One way in which siblings (in one instance, even a mother) in resource poor households manage to get extra food is by offering tidbits to the youngest child, then consuming the food when the youngest child "doesn't want it."

Food is also given as a reward and denied as a punishment. All households purchased sweets (hard candies, crackers, gum) by the piece to appease or reward children. Some mothers planned ahead and bought and sequestered candies in bulk. They then doled out individual pieces for lower expense and effort than if they had bought loose sweets at a local store. Alternatively, children might be rewarded for completing tasks with coins that were usually converted within minutes to candies or breads. Buying older children's cooperation and younger children's silence with sweets, then, was a significant way in which working mothers got through the day with minimal interference from children.

Again, parents varied in how skillfully they distributed limited resources to keep all well fed. The most vulnerable individuals were the children just removed from the breast or replaced in the favored position of youngest child. Such youngsters suffered both the psychological deprivation of becoming ex-favorites and the material deprivation of no longer receiving the choicest tidbits. Additionally, they were unable to compete with older siblings at the family pot—although in this culture the food preparer ordinarily dished out the individual portions.

RELATIONSHIP OF MOTHERS' INCOME TO FOOD

In contrast to fathers' income, which, where present, went into meeting general household expenses, mothers' income, if separate from general household income, went directly into food purchases. In tortilla households women went to the market and sold tortillas. They then immediately purchased the maize for the next day's tortillas and spent what was left over on the day's food supplies and on any other sundries they thought necessary. Although their purchases also included such nonfood items as crockery, flowers, candles, or animal feed at times, the bulk of their income went directly to food purchases. In households where women kept accounts separate from their husbands' (rather than pooling general family income, as household #2), their money was spent for food and other household expenses; men's income went to household construction, services, and large expenses. Men also invested in trade and, sometimes, in improving their capital technology (they purchased weaving looms or sewing machines, for example). Even where women got the bulk of their household money from men, whatever extra money they earned went to meet food expenses.

Alternatively, women's income from crafts or trade could be

used to buy time from food processing for their own households, particularly tortilla making. Deciding whether to make tortillas— the major "filling" food of the diet—was very deliberate. It took into account the drudgery involved (buying the maize, carrying it home, putting up the *nixtamal* [maize kernels with limestone], washing the *nixtamal*, going to the mill, making the fire, making the tortillas); alternative uses of the woman's time; and the cost, but also the quality, of the tortillas that could be purchased. Women who needed extra time for sewing nevertheless got up at 6 A.M. to prepare tortillas for large families, since they felt that they could not purchase a product equivalent to the homemade tortillas in the marketplace. Also, preparing tortillas at home meant that less money in total was spent on the maize staple and on other foods, since people could fill up more cheaply and happily on the larger, tastier homemade tortillas and were therefore less hungry for other foods.

In contrast to reports on how middle-class women spend their incomes, there did not appear to be allocations by women to "pin money." Children are expected to contribute to the household budget; in return they receive food, care, clothing, and allowances. Each household works out its own arrangement: Some of the children work at home, others work outside the house and therefore have more autonomy in controlling their income allocation. Young women, for example, may want to purchase clothes, makeup, or just spend money on a good time with their friends. But such expenses are a source of contention with the mother, who wants the money to meet household expenses. What may be equally important for the family food budget is that daughters are available to aid the mother in her homemaking and child care tasks, and therefore help her improve her earnings, which improves the quantity and quality of the diet.

OTHER HOUSEHOLD FACTORS RELATED TO WOMEN'S ACTIVITIES AND DIET

Childhood illnesses and sanitation were two other factors affecting women's time and the diets of household members. Respiratory infections, diarrhea, and vomiting were the most frequent child-hood illnesses reducing appetite, food intake, and growth of patients. The drain on the mother's time and energies was considerable. Up to 50 percent of some mothers' time might be spent in child care if the youngest were ill, about twice her normal time allocation to child care. Even more upsetting for her was that the illnesses were often beyond her control. In situations where children played in extended family compounds, *all* children and grounds had to be kept sanitary or any child had a chance of picking up infections. One mother's boiling of all bottles, sanitary preparation of all foods, careful laundering of all clothing with soap and hot water, and assiduous removal of feces and other sources of contamination from her immediate yard still could not keep her children from illness, if, for example, they played in an extended family compound littered with the feces of others. In such cases, efforts at good nutrition and sound health practices are in vain—the children suffer illness anyway.

The methodological choice to follow women in households over twelve-hour periods, supplemented by opportunistic visits, also showed great variability in patterns of women's time allocation, both from household to household and within households on different days. Time spent working for monetary reimbursement, for instance, varied from 2 percent to 24 percent daily within individual households, and from 2 percent to 50 percent between households across days. Child care, which was analyzed as primary (when no other task was being performed) or secondary (if it did not interfere with another activity, such as food preparation or cash work), varied from 10 percent to 50 percent, depending on the household and the particular day of observation. With regard to work, there were full days and empty days whose scheduling affected food provisioning. Festivals, life-cycle events, and school duties all interrupted cash work and directly and indirectly affected the diet of other household members. Finally, food acquisition and consumption choices, although embedded in other economic concerns, were always a principal consideration of the focal woman. To "get through the day" meant meeting the responsibility of providing the two main meals. Although they might arrange their meal preparations and selections around their need for time to complete cash work, the day was complete only when everyone had been fed their expected meals.

CONCLUSIONS

The preceding sections highlight some of the interrelationships between women's work, child care, and dietary planning. In general, women in this culture work to provide food money, even if there is another earner or earners in the household. How much time they have to carry out cash work and still care for their households depends on the material conditions of production (especially whether they have a gas or petroleum stove and running water) and women's skills in organizing other available household labor to perform cash-earning and domestic tasks. There is no simple relationship between women's income, their time expenditure, and nutrient intake. In Mitla, the poorest households eat fewer meals and ingest fewer nutrients each day than those that are better off. In such households, women's income does not necessarily lead to well-nourished children, whether measured by nutrient intake or by anthropometric standards. Even where women work, they may be unable to reverse the truism that malnutrition is associated with poverty. Many variables enter into the ways women perform even such standard tasks as food preparation. In this setting, it would be difficult to set up an experiment to test the hypothesis that women who suffer deficits in nutrient intake (in contrast to others who are adequately nourished according to the same international nutrition standard) spend significantly less time working, more time resting, and produce significantly less. The availability of other resources, and how a woman manages them, intervene.

More positively, however, women's income in all cases was put directly into the food budget, sometimes toward the purchase of specific foods, such as milk, so that children might benefit. Moreover, the data did not indicate that the children of working mothers suffered poor hygiene or poorer diets as a result of the mothers' putting time into production for market rather than into home care. Meals might be delayed, but they were no lower in nutrient content; and extra cash meant that there were snacks to tide children over between meals. Nutrition policy attention to the nutritional quality of these snack foods might further enhance their dietary benefit.

An additional question is that of illness in relation to housework and eating patterns in the main social unit and the location where they sleep, eat, and play. This study has shown that children "eat around"; that they pick up infections "around"; and that in the first case positive effects, in the second case negative ones stem from residential patterns beyond the nuclear household. Mothers (and parents more generally, where both parents worked at home) fitted in productive activities around the demands for child care when the children were ill.

Finally, in future projects, investigators should take care to establish what weekly consumption and production cycles are, what typical daily consumption patterns are over this cycle, and calculate not only one- or three-day nutrient intakes but the nutrient intake over the entire cycle. In retrospect, it would have been beneficial to have had weekly cycles of meals and activities, rather than the two-day sequences in two different seasons: The combination of observations and interviews established that food consumption and cash production often move in weekly (rather than two-day) cycles, with periods of full time and empty time and periods of high quality protein consumption versus minimal protein intake. People who appear on certain days in a cycle to be underconsuming, yet not losing weight, may be making up energy deficits at another point in the cycle. It would also be desirable to show how activity patterns and related energy expenditures adjust or remain the same over days with small but significant differences in energy intakes; that is, whether people's work pacing changes according to daily food intakes where nutrient intake shows regular daily variations within a cycle of time.

Anthropologists and others would do well to study these aspects of diet, household organization and "mothercraft," and snacking behaviors of children (rather than simply dietary intake in relation to "family" factors) if they wish to learn why some households succeed and others fail nutritionally under environmental conditions that appear to be the "same."

NOTES

Acknowledgments: The research for this chapter was supported by a Social Science Research Council Latin American and Caribbean Area Advanced Individual Research Grant, "Mitla, Oaxaca, Mexico in Ten Year Perspective," June 1980–May 1981. The chapter was revised while the author was a Fellow at the Center for Advanced Study in the Behavioral Sciences, Stanford, California. I am grateful for the support of National Science Foundation Grant BNS 76-22943. An earlier version of my study was presented at the symposium "Diet and Domestic Organization" at the American Anthropological Association Annual Meeting, December 1981, in Los Angeles, California.

1. Households are coresidential units whose members, usually related by kinship, share common consumption and production tasks. The practice of virilocal residence, whereby sons are given lots from their father's household land to construct independent households, leads to the formation of household compounds, where members of several households, related by blood, while residing in separate buildings and eating from their own family pots, often share a common yard.

2. Criteria for selection included ages and numbers of children, occupational characteristics, and willingness of households to cooperate. Since the recording technique meant that a trained observer stayed with a household for entire days (twelve or thirteen hours), not all households immediately agreed to participate, although I received only one direct rebuff. The sample might be seen, however, as skewed (1) toward households of limited means, who seemed to enjoy the attention and prestige an observer's presence conferred, since the observer also visited regularly (though without prior announcement) on other occasions to check that activity patterns she had observed were indeed routine, and (2) away from wealthier households, who wished to keep their business transactions private.

3. The time-descriptive diary method also provided data on qualitative characteristics of interactions between mothers and children, fathers and children, and men and women. Descriptions included some indications of the "density" of work performance, an aspect of "work" usually missed by other methods of timed activity recording (see Erasmus 1980).

T A B L E   3.1
Household Characteristics

Household Composition	Occupations	House and Sanitary Facilities	Cooking	Meals
#1 Mo (pregnant)	Tortillas, sews, crochets	Adobe	Wood fire	One to two/day (vegetarian), plus one coffee
Fa	Weaves, wage labor	Backyard		
S, 14	[Weaves]			
D, 11	[Tortillas]			
S, 7				
D, 5				
S, 2				
#2 Mo	Tortillas, chocolate	Adobe, concrete	Gas stove	Two/day (one vegetarian), plus one coffee
Fa	Weaves, trades textiles, etc.	Toilet, shower		
D, 28	Tortillas, chocolate, dolls			
D, 25	Tortillas, cuts and sews, machine embroiders			
S, 18	Weaves			
D, 14	Tortillas, food processing			
S, 13	Weaves			
Gs,13	Weaves			
S, 11	Weaves			

T A B L E 3.1 *(continued)*

Household Composition	Occupations	House and Sanitary Facilities	Cooking	Meals
#3 Mo	Sews	Adobe	Gas stove	Two/day (one
Fa	Weaves	Latrine		vegetarian), plus
D, 12	Sews			one coffee
S, 10	[Weaves]			
S, 8				
D, 5				
D, 2				
#4 Mo	Macrame, crochets, tortillas	Adobe	Gas stove	Two/day
Fa	Agriculture, wage work	Backyard		(vegetarian), plus
S, 18	Agriculture, trades			two coffees
S, 15	Agriculture			
D, 11	Tortillas			
D, 5				
D, 1				
#5 Mo	Tortillas, sews, crochets	Adobe	Petroleum	Two/day (one
Fa	Sews, sells ices	Backyard		vegetarian), plus
D, 11	Crochets, [tortillas]			one coffee
S, 8				
S, 4				
D, ½				

#6	Gmo		Adobe	Wood fire	One to two/day (vegetarian)
	Mo	Tortillas, macrame, laundry, crochets	Backyard		
	D, 12	Tortillas, macrame, laundry, crochets			
	D, 6	Tortillas, laundry, crochets			
	S, 1				
#7	Mo	Sews, trades, crochets	Plaster	Gas stove	Two/day (one vegetarian), plus two coffees
	Fa	Mason			
	D, 9				
	D, 8				
	D, 5				
	D, 2				
#8	Mo (Pregnant)	Sews, dolls	Plaster	Gas stove	Two/day (one vegetarian), plus two coffees
	Fa	Weaves			
	D, 16	Studies, sews, dolls			
	S, 14	Studies, weaves			
	S, 12	[Weaves]			
	S, 10	[Weaves]			
	S, 8	[Weaves]			
	S, 6				
	S, 4				
	D, 2				

T A B L E 3.1 (*continued*)

Household Composition	Occupations	House and Sanitary Facilities	Cooking	Meals
#9 Mo (pregnant)	Sews	Adobe	Gas stove	Two/day
Fa	Sews	Backyard		
S, 13	Sews			
S, 11				
S, 9				
S, 2				
#10 Mo (pregnant)	Trades	Adobe	Gas stove	Two/day (one vegetarian)
Fa	Dolls, weaves, trade	Backyard		
S, 7				
S, 5				
S, 2				
#11 Mo (pregnant)	Tortillas, dolls	Adobe	Wood platform	Two/day (vegetarian), plus one coffee
Fa	Mason	Backyard		
D, 6				
S, 4				
D, 2				
#12 Mo	Tortillas, chocolate	Adobe	Wood platform	Two/day (vegetarian)
Fa	Agriculture, firewood	Backyard		

#13 Mo — Sews
Fa — Weaves
S, 6
D, 5
S, 2
Adobe / Backyard — Wood fire — Two/day (vegetarian)

#14 Mo — Sews
Fa — Weaves, agriculture
S, 17 — Dolls, cuts and sews, trades
S, 15 — Weaves
S, 12 — Weaves
S, 9
D, 6
S, 4
Adobe / Backyard — Gas stove — Two/day (one vegetarian), plus one coffee

#15 Mo — [Crochets]
Fa — Musician, electrician
S, 4
S, 3
S, 2
S, ½
Adobe / Backyard — Gas stove — Two/day (one vegetarian)

#16 Mo (pregnant) — Sews, crochets
Fa — Weaves
D, 3
D, 1
Adobe / Backyard — Petroleum — Two/day (vegetarian)

T A B L E 3.1 *(continued)*

Household Composition	Occupations	House and Sanitary Facilities	Cooking	Meals
#17 Gmo	Sews, shopkeeps	Adobe	Gas stove	Two/day, plus
Mo	Sews, shopkeeps	Backyard		two coffees
D, 6				
D, 4				
D, 2				
#18 Female	Cuts and sews	Abode	Wood fire	Two/day, plus
		Backyard		one coffee
#19 Mo	Cuts and sews	Plaster	Gas stove	Two/day,
Fa	Trades	Backyard		plus milk
S, 2				
S, 1				
#20 Mo	Trades	Adobe	Gas stove	Two/day,
Fa	Weaves, trades	Backyard		plus snacks
D, 5				
D, 3				

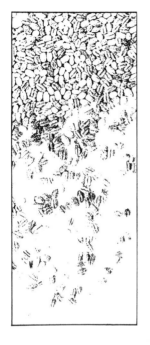

Impact of Health on Women's Food-Procurement Strategies on a Guatemalan Plantation

Mary Scrimshaw

Sheila Cosminsky

Nutritional anthropologists generally focus on food, diet, and nutritional status, illness and health being considered primarily as they directly affect nutrient intake, nutrient availability and absorption, and nutritional status. Other medical anthropologists study illness, disease, and the use of different curers and health care services. What Mary Scrimshaw and Sheila Cosminsky have initiated with their work is a more synthetic approach to analyzing the interrelations between diet, nutrition, illness, and treatment. In doing so, they focus on food acquisition and the pathways by which food enters the household, in a way reminiscent of parts of Lewin's (1943) channel theory. Women are seen as the main "gatekeepers" (although men, and sometimes children, make important contributions), and they are the ones whose activities are most closely analyzed. Scrimshaw and Cosminsky show the many ways in which the health of women, men, and children bears on the acquisition, distribution, and use of food and income. They demonstrate also how people's perceptions of illness and available treatment affect domestic activities, food provisioning, and the health and survival of all household members.

Since they carried out their work on a Guatemalan coffee–sugar plantation, their study also provides a particularly clear and graphic example of how organization of labor for production for the international commodity market can have far-reaching and detrimental effects on the domestic organization, health, and nutrition of employees and their families. They show how men are more rigidly constrained by the plantation organization and how, in their permanently precarious situation, women seek, in changing and flexible ways, to ensure that their households have food and remedies for illness.

Food procurement involves all activities by which food enters the household, including earning income, exchanging commodities, purchasing, gathering, and processing, as well as producing food. Women play a critical role in this process, which requires managerial and decision-making skills and a thorough knowledge of the physical and social environment. This chapter analyzes women's role in food procurement on a Guatemalan coffee and sugar plantation and the impact of health and illness on their ability to perform.

Dewalt (1983; Dewalt, Kelly, and Pelto 1980) has focused on alternative dietary or nutritional strategies and on the multiple pathways by which food enters households in relation to income and to their implications for dietary adequacy. Little attention has been paid, however, to the effect that the health and nutritional status of women and their families have on women's food behavior and on their ability to provision their families adequately. In this chapter we show the profound impact that health and illness, of both the women and their families, have on their food procuring strategies and how they influence the allocation of time, energy, and cash. We explore economic position, seasonality, household organization, and relationships between kin as factors that also affect food procuring strategies. The interplay or interaction of these factors is illustrated through the use of case studies.

SETTING

The research was carried out on Finca San Felipe (pseudonym), a family-owned sugar and coffee plantation (*finca*)[1] located on the Pacific coast of Guatemala. Finca San Felipe covers an area of 1,384 acres, placing it in the top 2 percent of farms in the country by size. It has a resident population of about seven hundred, of mixed Mayan and Ladino[2] heritage, consisting mainly of second- and third-generation Mayan migrants from different towns in the Western highlands. Land, labor, and housing are controlled and allocated by the plantation owner (*finquero*).

The finca is a compact community of approximately 116 households. Most, though not all, houses are adjacent, single large rooms about twelve feet by eighteen feet in area (which may be subdivided by their inhabitants), in long, multiple-room dwelling units with wood walls, dirt floors, and tin roofs. People live in close proximity to each other and households are linked through kinship, affinal, and other ties. In general, housing is poor and overcrowded. Drinking water is supplied primarily by four public taps, while the streams are used for washing and bathing. Latrines are almost nonexistent, except in a few homes of salaried workers. Most households are nuclear or two generational. The average household size is 5.6 persons, although households range from large three-generation families (with as many as thirteen inhabitants) at one extreme (those living in large, separate housing units), to single-person households at the other (Cosminsky and Scrimshaw 1981).

Food Use and Purchase

Food use by the people of the finca follows the traditional Meso-American pattern of corn and beans as staple foods. Tomatoes, onions, chili peppers, and herbs are made into *chirmols* or sauces that add flavor to tortillas, the form in which corn is most often consumed. Greens and vegetables are added to stews with meat or fish when available. White cheese and eggs are favorite lunch items if cash permits. Nontraditional foods include wheat bread, noodles, and dried soups (used as stew bases) and "Protemas," a dried precooked cottonseed flour and corn mixture enriched with B vitamins and iron. These are all popular because of ease of preparation.

Three meals a day is the basic pattern: *desayuno* (breakfast), *almuerzo* (lunch), and *cena* or *comida* (supper). Tortillas are eaten at every meal, accompanied by greens, beans, chili, soup or stew, cheese, eggs, or meat, depending on availability and affordability. The only distinction among the three meals is that coffee is usually drunk in the morning. Men and teenagers will often take their lunch with them to work; they prefer one of the foods that is both high status and high protein, such as meat, eggs, or cheese.

Men may also take a flask of *atol de maiz*, a thick corn drink, with them to the field and drink it between meals. Women and children may drink some *atol* (when available) around 10:00 A.M. but avoid it in the afternoon, as it is regarded as too heavy. On Saturdays, if finances permit, *tamales* (a special steamed dish made from corn dough and pieces of meat or beans, wrapped in banana or other special leaves), which cost $.05 each, are eaten.

The most popular snack foods (*galgeras*), consumed mainly by adolescents and children, are sugar flavored ices and packaged corn chips (*tortrix*). Traditional snack foods made from mangoes, *jocotes*, plaintains, watermelon flavored with squash seeds (*pepitoria*), and chili are sold locally on payday. Except for these snacks, few fruits are bought, but mangoes, bananas, papayas, and other fruits are gathered locally.

Sweetened coffee is the main drink consumed daily. Corn atoles are popular and are also used for special occasions. Soft drinks and beer are bought occasionally. Gaseous mineral water is used mainly as a medicinal drink. *Aguardiente* (*"guaro"*), the local alcoholic drink, is consumed heavily on payday by men and a few women and is always imbibed on ceremonial occasions by both men and women.

The finca is located one and a half hours' walk from the town of San Felipe and 12.5 kilometers from the departmental capital of Retalhuleu. Women usually make purchases only once or twice in a two-week period (*quincena*) at these nearby market towns. Some food is also purchased from six small stores on the plantation, from traveling food vendors, and from other finca women.

Health and Health Care

According to the finca surveys, general health status of the finca community is poor, with high morbidity and mortality rates. The people usually use home remedies as a first resort for health care. If this is not successful, they commonly buy patent remedies and pharmaceuticals from local stores, lay practitioners, or pharmacies. A variety of folk practitioners, both on and off the finca, are popu-lar. These include *curanderos* (curers), herbalists, spiritists, lay injectionists, and traveling vendors. Some formal or Western health care resources, such as health centers, physicians, and hospitals, which are located in the nearby towns, are also used (Cosminsky and Scrimshaw 1980; Cosminsky 1987).

METHODOLOGY

The data were obtained as part of a multidisciplinary longitudinal study of the nutritional and health status of the finca population carried out at intervals between 1970 and 1979. This chapter is based mainly on information collected in 1978, as part of a study focusing on women's productive and reproductive strategies and the allocation of resources between food and medicine. A sample of thirty-five households was selected for intensive interviewing and observation. Each household had at least two children, one of whom was under two years of age. The households were selected to represent a range of nutritional and health statuses as measured in previous studies on the finca.

Starting with market day, the "market basket" (food brought home) was analyzed, and the households were revisited at least three times a week for two-week periods, to check on all food items entering the households and on other patterns of expenditures. Detailed information was obtained on who buys or procures what, from where, and how (credit or cash or exchange). For the same two-week period, illness episodes and health seeking behavior were tabulated for all members of the family. Three or four two-week periods were studied: May through June, when cash and corn were scarce; July through August, the time of early harvest but low cash; and October, the peak season, when both cash and corn were plentiful. The October sample was a subsample of twelve households selected from the previous samples. The two-week period was chosen to coincide with the finca pay schedule of two weeks. Interviews were held with the administrative personnel of the finca and the finca records were used to obtain information about wages.

PROVISIONING SOURCES

The major sources of household provisioning are food crops produced on family plots (*milpas*) and cash from formal employment,
both controlled by the finca owner.

Subsistence Production

Each male worker (depending on his status as salaried employee,
permanent worker, or temporary worker) is provided with a small
plot of land from four to eight *cuerdas* (625 square meters), which
is used for subsistence crops of corn and beans. Tomatoes, greens,
and squash are also frequently grown. The whole family works on
the *milpa*, planting, maintaining, and harvesting. Men always plant
the corn; women usually plant the beans. Women and children do
most of the weeding and harvest early corn and vegetables. The
entire household works together to harvest the main crops.

There are two corn and bean harvests during the year. The
first, in July and August, brings the largest corn yield of approximately $10.71 a *cuerda*.[3] The second, in December and January, is
of about $4.22 a *cuerda* cash value. The *milpas* provide an impor-
tant but not sufficient proportion of the household's food and must
be supplemented by purchased food. Some families must buy corn
and beans from as early as April until July; all families buy these
staples for a portion of this period. Cash employment is essential
for an adequate food supply.

Formal Employment

Adults and children above fourteen years of age work as wage laborers on Finca San Felipe and sometimes on neighboring plantations. Men work year round in sugar and coffee production; most
(97) as *ganadores* (temporary workers who may be laid off two or
three months a year, at which time they seek work at other fincas);
some (54) as *colonos* (permanent workers who are guaranteed full-
time work); and a few (8) as *meseros* (salaried employees, such as

the office manager and the carpenter). *Ganadores* who were heads of households worked most of the year and were not laid off during 1976–78. Average earnings for men (whether *ganador* or *colono*) in 1978 during May was $18.00 a *quincena*; during October, $32.00 a *quincena*.

Women's cash work opportunities and amounts earned were highly variable. During most of the year there is little paid work for women on Finca San Felipe. A few women work irregularly drying sugarcane or in the coffee nurseries. Some women who do not have child-rearing responsibilities work on nearby fincas, where they may earn from $3.00 to $12.00 a *quincena*. All women, however, work as coffee pickers during the coffee season, mid August through November (115 were listed on the finca wage records as temporary workers.) Women, especially when picking with the help of their children, can double their earnings during the peak months of September and October. At this time they earned an average of $15.00 a *quincena*, and a few with children earned as much as $40.00.

Adolescents, working on nearby fincas, usually were paid one-half of an adult man's wage. They reported receiving varying amounts, most frequently $5.00 to $10.00 a *quincena*. The importance of women's and children's contributions is shown by the percentage of total household wage income they provide. As a minimal estimate, women sixteen years and older contribute an average of 17.7 percent, and children under sixteen contribute 15.1 percent, for a combined 32.8 percent of the total household wage income (Cosminsky and Scrimshaw 1981).

OPTIONS AND STRATEGIES
TO EXTEND RESOURCE BASE

The finca system organizes and controls the labor in the formal employment sector. However, wages from plantation employment and crops from the *milpa* are often not sufficient to provision a household adequately. Men are constrained by mandatory labor on the finca. They must work in the sugarcane fields and in the coffee groves (*cafetal*) during the peak coffee season. This, combined with working their *milpas*, takes most of their time and energy. Most entrepreneurial activities are perceived by the finca owner as conflicting with their responsibilities to him.

In contrast, women are temporary laborers who pick coffee and dry sugarcane waste (*bagazo*) in season. They have a more flexible obligatory work schedule, and their entrepreneurial activities are not seen as threatening to the finca system. When more wage labor on the finca is not available, they have looked to other means of augmenting their income and resources (Cosminsky and Scrimshaw 1981). Women, therefore, more often than men, give their time, energy, and skills to extending the resource base of their households.

Gathering Wild Foods

Several types of greens are gathered from nearby fields and hillsides (*monte*).[4] Seasonal fruits, including *jocotes*, mangoes, and *cushin*, are found in the nearby fields, plaintains and palm fruits in the coffee groves. The latter are an important source of food for animals. Coffee beans are sometimes taken from the ground during the picking season. Fish, shellfish, and eels are netted seasonally. A few men hunt or trap small game animals, such as armadillos, iguanas, squirrels, and birds.

Home Gardening and Animal Husbandry

Many families have small home gardens in which fruits, vegetables, and herbs may be grown. Pigs, chickens, turkeys, or ducks are raised by some women in these same patios. Animal husbandry provides a way for women to both expand their food supply and obtain some cash. Chickens and turkeys and their eggs may be eaten by the family on special occasions but are often sold for needed cash. Pigs are regarded mainly as an investment, but the time, work, and resources involved, together with the risk that they may die before the investment is realized, deter many women from raising them.

Marketing

Petty trading and food vending are important means by which women may obtain small but significant amounts of additional cash. Five women who own or whose husbands own cows make and sell cheese. Several other women cook and sell tamales on weekends to other finca families. A few women sell homemade snacks outside their homes on payday and on special occasions or at soccer games. Some women either bring their own fruits or buy fruits for resale in a nearby market town. Conversely, women may buy items in the market for resale on the finca.

For women who can obtain the initial capital, small stores are a favored entrepreneurial activity (Cosminsky and Scrimshaw 1981). Of the six on the finca, five are managed by women, the sixth by a disabled man. "*Guaro*" (a sugar-based alcoholic drink produced and marketed clandestinely) is sold locally by a number of families.

Providing Services

A few women sew clothing for finca clients. The demand for clothing varies and is greatest at the opening of the school year, with the need for school uniforms, and at Easter.

Curing is another means of earning income. There are two midwives on the finca who not only assist at childbirth but also give advice to women on health and other problems. They charge between $5 and $10 a birth and for consultations. There are several traditional practitioners, or curers (*curanderos*), on the finca, of whom five are women. They often specialize in children's illnesses, such as the evil eye, and receive a small amount of cash or gifts as payment. There are two female injectionists, who charge for giving injections and one woman who sells and gives advice on Western medicines (Cosminsky and Scrimshaw 1980).

Other Food Sources

Other sources of food include gifts, food exchanges, free food, and rations.

Gifts and Exchanges. The activation and use of kin ties, not only within a household but also between households, is important in expanding one's resource base. Food may be given as gifts or exchanged for other food. Younger people might help out elderly parents, or parents might help children in difficulty. Young children may receive snacks from grandparents or godparents.

More common than gifts are favors that involve food. For example, a woman who has pigs will give preference to kin to raise them, or, if someone kills a pig, close kin will have first pick of the meat or may buy some at a lower price. Siblings, parents, and children will also help each other by buying for each other at the market, especially in case of illness. Food transfers also occur when workers share their lunches.

In addition to these everyday exchanges, others occur at such special and ritual occasions as Easter, weddings, and funerals, when households share food with their neighbors, as well as with kin.

Free Food and Rations. Several women receive flour, oil, and powdered milk monthly from the public health clinic in San Felipe and from the Catholic church, through programs for mothers with infants. In order to be registered in the clinic food program, women must have gone to the prenatal clinic during their pregnancy and must attend a nutrition class. The time and inconvenience involved in obtaining and preparing the food, as well as its erratic availability, make this an unreliable and unpopular food source. Powdered milk is often said to taste *"feo"* (ugly) without white sugar and may not be consumed without it.

Salaried workers (*meseros*) receive rations of brown sugar (*panela*), corn, and firewood. Full-time workers (*colonos*) are sometimes given or sometimes sold rations of coffee and brown sugar at reduced prices. Brown sugar is considered inferior to white sugar, and the rations may be sold. Temporary workers (*ganadores*) do not receive any rations.

Management of Cash and Other Resources

Women are responsible for managing the household budget and make most food purchases, except for corn (and sometimes sugar) provided by men. The female household head keeps and controls all of the cash that she earns, together with that contributed by other household and family members. Men are expected to contribute part of their earnings toward general expenses, and adolescents twelve to fourteen are expected to give the major portion of their earnings to their mother. Some adolescent girls and young unmarried women work as domestics in Guatemala City and send remittances. Women also organize children's work activities, both for earning cash and for procuring food directly.

Another strategy women use for maximizing their cash, or for obtaining goods when cash is short, is to modify their purchasing practices. Although buying food in town markets is cheaper in the long run, it necessitates purchasing larger quantities and using time and energy in travel. When money, time, and energy are in short supply, women may choose to shop locally, where they can buy in smaller quantities and on credit. Obtaining credit is a critical aspect of a woman's economic strategies, as is borrowing (from kin, godparents, neighbors, finca owners, and moneylenders) in emergencies or during hard times.

HEALTH AND NUTRITIONAL STATUS

The options and strategies discussed above emphasize the critical role women play in the process of food provisioning. Several factors constrain them from optimally carrying out this role. One of the most important but least examined of these is their own health status and that of their families.

Surveys done on the finca in 1970, 1972, and 1976 show that the general health and nutritional status of the population is poor. Although most frequent in young children, diarrheal and respiratory infections are common at all ages. A number of adults had active or treated tuberculosis. The high frequency of decayed or missing teeth, periodontal disease, and dental abscesses further contributed to ill health.

Morbidity from infectious disease varied widely among households, but one-half of the population had more than three episodes per household, and one-fourth described more than five in the two-week period covered by the morbidity interview. The prevalence of acute diseases varies with the season: Diarrheal illnesses increase with the onset of the rainy season, and respiratory diseases are most common during the dry season, although both are hyperendemic. Iron deficiency anemia, resulting from the low amount of iron in the diet and blood loss from hookworm, was frequent in all age groups. There is now good evidence that these conditions result in reduced physical capacity, impaired immunity, increased infectious disease, and adverse effects on cognitive performance. Even iron deficiency not severe enough to cause anemia can have these consequences.

Women's Health

At least 70 percent of the women between twenty and thirty years of age are either pregnant, lactating, or both (Cosminsky and Scrimshaw 1981). Moreover, lactation most commonly continues for two years. This places a heavy biological demand on the woman, including increased need for calories and essential nutrients. The food intake of women differs somewhat from that of men. Women consumed meat, eggs, and cheese less frequently and their servings were smaller; however, they did eat more greens and other vegetables. A dietary survey showed that the calorie and protein intakes of lactating women on the finca were only 80 percent of WHO recommended allowances and that those of vitamin A and niacin were less than 75 percent (Peck 1970). In a 1976 survey only 8 percent of pregnant women and none of the lactating women were meeting the recommended dietary level for calories (Gilbert 1976). Reduction of physical activity would have been essential to achieve energy balance on these low intakes.

Pregnancy and lactation in themselves may not affect food procurement, because women continue to work during these periods. However, the effect of such low nutrient intakes on their health and immune status may precipitate more illness episodes and create an energy deficit, thus constraining their food- and cash-procuring activities. Various gynecological problems, among them vaginal bleeding and "fallen uterus" (*decompostura*), were mentioned by several women as interfering with their activities to obtain food and cash.

Men's Health

Illness of the male household head affects family food intake primarily through his absence from work and loss of income. Alcohol is a major factor influencing the health and nutritional state not only of men but also of the rest of the household. Although we do not have quantitative data, there is no doubt that a significant proportion of some men's wages is spent on alcohol. Drinking not only takes away money from the household budget and food supply but may also result in inability to work, especially the day after payday, and thus reduces wages. Households in which men consumed a large quantity of alcohol were also usually ones with poor health and nutrition records. Project surveys showed a higher prevalence of anemia among men than women. This may have stemmed from more drinking (or more exposure to hookworm) among men. Men's lower intake of greens may also have contributed to iron deficiency or anemia.

Children's Health

A survey made on the finca in 1970 showed that children eighteen to thirty-six months of age were consuming less than 75 percent of the recommended allowance for calories, protein, calcium, niacin, and vitamin A. Associated with this is significantly retarded growth and development, indicating protein–energy malnutrition. In 1976, an anthropometric survey using the Gomez method of classification demonstrated that of 113 children studied 40 (35 percent) were found to have second-degree malnutrition (60–74 percent of standard weight for age) and 4 (.04 percent) had third-degree malnutrition (less than 60 percent of standard weight for age). Diarrheal diseases and respiratory infections are the most frequent diseases among children. Skin and eye infections are common. Communicable childhood diseases, measles, and whooping cough occur epidemically and may lead to serious complications or death.

CASE STUDIES

Case studies bring into relief the dynamics and complex interrelationships among the various factors that affect food provisioning. The case studies that follow have been selected to represent different illness situations and the impact such health factors have on women's food acquisition behavior and thus the family food supply. These situations include chronic illness of both the woman and members of her family, acute illness, and alcoholism.[5]

Case Study A: Elena

This case study illustrates the effect of the chronic ill health of the mother and the rest of the members of the household, especially an infant, on the food provisioning of a young nuclear family with a high dependency ratio.

Elena is a twenty-seven-year-old mother with four small children, ranging in age from one to ten years. Her husband, Antonio, is a *ganador* and the only full-time wage earner. Everyone in the family was sick for most of the study period. At various times Elena had fever, chills, sore throat, cough and swollen glands, diarrhea, stomach cramps, and urinary bleeding. All the children suffered on and off from colds, cough, fevers, and diarrhea. Miguel, the baby, was the sickest, with diarrhea, vomiting, fever sores, and conjunctivitis.

In this period the family spent at least $67.00, seeking help from the public health clinic, private physicians, injectionists, shamans, and spiritists, and using a variety of herbs, patent remedies, pharmaceuticals, injections, prayers, and rituals.

During the lean season from April through July, Antonio, the father, had an average income of $17.00 a *quincena*. In order to buy medicine and meat, they sold corn several times. Sometimes this meant selling the corn for $.08 a pound, two cents below the market rate. Starting in June, they had to buy corn. During one *quincena* in July (when Antonio had earned only $14.00 because he had been sick), after paying the $11.00 that they owed for corn, Elena and Antonio had only $3.00 left for all other food. They did

T A B L E 4.1
Money Spent for Important Food Items:
Case Study A, Elena, Finca San Felipe, Guatemala, 1978
(Household size—6; consumption unit—4.4)

Food	May	June	July	October
Corn	milpa	milpa	$11.00 (100 lbs.)	milpa
Meat	$1.50 (3 lbs.)	$.50 (1 lb.)	.55 (1 lb.)	$3.90 (8 lbs.)
Fish	—	—	.60 (1 lb.)	1.95 (3 lbs.)
Eggs	.10	—	—	—
Cheese	—	.30	1.50	.90
Beans	2.10 (7 lbs.)	.70 (2 lbs.)	milpa	6.60 (21 lbs.)
Sugar				
White	2.08 (16 lbs.)	.60 (3 lbs.)	—	1.06 (7 lbs.)
Brown	—	3.00	2.00	2.60
Rice	1.44 (6 lbs.)	.50 (2 lbs.)	.50 (2 lbs.)	2.80 (11 lbs.)
Pasta	.15 (½ lb.)	.30 (1 lb.)	.30 (1 lb.)	1.00 (3 lbs.)
Protemas	—	—	—	.30
Vegetables	.40	.35	.65	.98
Greens (gathered)	some	some	many	few
Animal protein per consumption unit*	.36	.18	.59	1.53

Note: Consumption units were calculated for each household. These were based on caloric requirements of the individuals in the household, calculated according to age and sex (using the 1973 FAO/WHO expert report on protein–energy requirements). The number of consumption units in a household is the sum of the number of calories required by each family member (FAO/WHO), divided by the average number of calories required by men on the finca aged 21 to 30 years. Since their weight averaged 54 kg. (119 pounds), this was approximately 2,500 calories.

*The cash spent for animal-protein foods (meat, fish, eggs, cheese, and milk) was calculated for each family. This factor, divided by the consumption unit, gives an indication of how well nutrient needs are met in households of different composition.

not buy any meat, beans, rice, or white sugar, and reduced their consumption of *panela* (brown sugar). During this period, Elena increased her gathering activities, substituting greens for other food. They ate greens of five different types at least eight times during a *quincena*.

Elena said that since she is frequently sick and the children are always sick, she has not been able to work like some of the other women or to go out and clean the fields. She said she was ashamed (*me da verguenza*) because they had nothing; they were poorer than many others and there was always sickness. "If there was no sickness, we would have some money, but since we are sick, there is none."

In August, they harvested the corn and sold a hundred pounds for $11.00, which they used for medical treatment for the baby. Later in August, Elena borrowed $10.00 from the plantation owner to pay off food and medical debts. This would be deducted from her pay during coffee-picking season in October.

By that month the situation had vastly improved. The baby was well. Elena was picking coffee and with the girls' help earned $20.00. Her husband earned $37.00 for the *quincena* October 14–27, more than double what he had been earning in July and August. He gave her $10.00 and paid off several of their debts. In addition, they had corn from their harvest. That *quincena*, Elena bought eight pounds of meat and three pounds of fish for $5.85, compared to one pound of meat she bought between May 28 and June 10 or July 23 and August 5 for $.55. She also bought twenty-one pounds of beans, compared to two pounds that she bought between May 28 and June 10 (see Table 4.1).

Case Study B: Teresa

This case study of a mature family illustrates how alcoholism and a woman's health problems result in severely reduced cash income.

Teresa's family represents a mature household with good income potential. Pedro (forty-nine years old) and Teresa (thirty-seven) live with their son Mario, his wife (Lucia), and four younger children. This family's finances, relationships, and problems are complex. Teresa had potential cash and resource help from two adult wage earners (Pedro, a full-time, and Mario, a temporary worker), one adolescent son, Roberto, together with an occasional remittance from a daughter, Marta, in Guatemala City.

Teresa's husband, however, drank excessively. He contributed corn but seldom provided money for the household budget. This problem, plus her own vaginal bleeding, and Mario's being hospitalized for "attacks" that were probably alcohol related, left her in a desperate spiral of food inadequacy and heavy debts.

Teresa had had vaginal bleeding and pain since March. She had tried several treatments in a nearby clinic and locally, running up debts of more than $16.00. The traditional midwife gave her a cure and told Teresa that she must rest for twenty days.

On April 29 (payday) Mario arrived home from work with violent vomiting, diarrhea, and shaking attacks. After some home remedies had proven unsuccessful, he was taken to the hospital in Retalhuleu, where he stayed for four days. Mario was able to return to work in six days, but food and cash were both scarce in the household. Pedro had paid off their corn and sugar debt of $15.00, but no money was left for other food. Mario's usual contribution of $8.00 for food all went for his medical bills.

Teresa was despondent. There was very little to eat in the house except corn, one small bunch of onions, a pound of tomatoes bought from a neighbor, and some greens that she and Roberto had picked in the *monte*. There were no beans and no rice (which, with corn, were considered staples), and nobody wanted to give her credit. She had gotten up early to make tortillas with *chirmol* for Roberto to take for lunch at work. Roberto, however, was lying on the bed; he had not gone to work because he was too embarrassed to bring only tortillas. Since the workers share their lunches, he must at least have beans, or, better, an egg, cheese, or a bit of meat for his friends. Teresa said that he would eat greens at home but never outside. For the next two weeks Roberto worked off and on with his mother in the *milpa*, and she collected several types of greens in the *monte* to augment their diet. Teresa sold some shoes for $6.00 and extended her credit, but by the end of

T A B L E   4.2
Money Spent for Important Food Items:
Case Study B, Teresa, Finca San Felipe, Guatemala, 1978
(Household size—8; consumption unit—6.7)

Food	May	July	October
Corn	$14.00 (140 lbs.)	milpa	milpa
Meat	5.38 (7 lbs.)	$4.35 (6½ lbs.)	$7.45
Eggs	.60 (1 doz.)	.60	2.10
Cheese	1.20	.60	.90
Beans	4.05 (11 lbs.)	3.65	5.34 (17 lbs.)
Sugar			
White	1.60	—	2.00 (12 lbs.)
Brown	—	ration (8 lbs.)*	—
Rice	.25 (1 lb.)	.48 (2 lbs.)	1.00 (4 lbs.)
Pasta	—	.30 (1 lb.)	.45 (1½ lbs.)
Protemas	.30 (1 lb.)	.30	.90 (2 lbs.)
Vegetables	.87	.55	.40
Greens			
(gathered)	some	some	none
Animal			
protein per			
consumption			
unit	1.07	.83	1.56

*Brown sugar was received as a ration from the finca owner.

the month she owed money to five local stores, two neighbors, and two curers.

By the end of July none of the storekeepers would give Teresa credit, and her neighbors refused to lend her more money. Pedro, her husband, contributed nothing for food, even though the finca office reported his earnings as $15.73 for that period. As their contribution to the family food budget, she received $8.00 from Mario, $6.00 from Roberto, and $4.00 from Marta, who had come home from the city to help out her ill mother. This money, however, had to be used for past debts as well as for that month's food.

To obtain more money for food, Pedro sold some *panela* to the midwife for $2.50, with which he bought beans, eggs, "protemas," oil, and rice. Mario's wife, Lucia, who had given birth to a girl, got some dried milk from the church. They did not use this either for the baby or for themselves, as was their intent, because they had no white sugar to add to it. Teresa sold their last pig to pay off medical debts.

By October, the peak season for cash from coffee picking and when *milpa* corn was plentiful, the family had recovered somewhat. Pedro bought twelve pounds of white sugar for $2.00 and paid $4.00 for a dress for their nine-year-old daughter because she had worked with him picking coffee. He gave no additional food money, though the finca reported his earnings as $22.86. Teresa, however, working with Roberto earned $41.60. Mario contributed $8.00 to the household. Marta gave nothing, because she was working off a debt to another finca. Teresa bought shoes and clothing for all the children, including Roberto, and paid off most of her debts. She bought more meat, eggs, beans, rice, pasta, and "protemas," though fewer vegetables, than in the previous *quincenas*, (see Table 4.2).

Case Study C: Delia

Delia exemplifies a woman who, when well, made good use of natural resources to augment her family's diet. Her acute illness so reduced her activities that she could no longer gather supplementary food for the family.

Delia, twenty-six, has an eight-year-old daughter, Guadalupe, by her first husband, whom she left because he drank too much. She has children of thirty months and eight months by her second husband, Juan, forty-seven, who is a *colono*. Juan drinks a lot on paydays and sometimes beats her when drunk, but she says he is responsible most of the time.

Delia did not have serious debt problems. She bought some eggs, cheese, sugar, and other food on credit from local stores but did not overextend her debts. The supply of corn was adequate for

T A B L E 4.3
Money Spent for Important Food Items:
Case Study C, Delia, Finca San Felipe, Guatemala, 1978
(Household size—5; consumption unit—3.5)

Food	May	July	October
Corn	milpa	$2.25 + milpa	milpa
Corn products (tamales)	—	.30	$ .75
Meat	$5.75 (9½ lbs.)	5.20 (6½ lbs.)	9.70 (10½ lbs.)
Fish	river (2 lbs.)	—	1.40 (3 lbs.)
Eggs	1.60 (20)	1.74 (24)	1.60 (20)
Cheese	1.80	1.20	1.80
Beans	1.20 (4 lbs.)	1.20 (4 lbs.)	1.80 (6 lbs.)
Sugar White	1.81 (12 lbs.)	.16 (1 lb.)	1.28 (8 lbs.)
Brown	—	—	—
Rice	.25 (1 lb.)	.75 (3 lbs.)	.50 (2 lbs.)
Pasta	.16 (½ lb.)	.16 (½ lb.)	.16 (½ lb.)
Protemas	—	—	—
Vegetables	1.55	1.95	1.25
Greens (gathered)	many	few	many
Animal protein per consumption unit	2.60	2.30	4.10

a young family. As a *colono*, Juan received eight *cuerdas* of *milpa*, and theirs is one of the few households that has a metal storage bin for corn, preventing loss of grain to rats. In June, Delia sold four pounds of corn to buy some sugar and bread, along with snacks for the children.

Delia also did not run up large medical debts. In June, she treated her children's diarrhea with Enterolan, which she bought in a pharmacy for $1.09, and treated their colds with Vicks, which

costs $.05. For her own medical problems, when home herbal treat-
ment did not suffice, she usually went to a doctor in Retalhuleu,
who charged $4.00 an illness episode and often gave free medi-
cines.

Delia liked greens and enjoyed fishing. She customarily augmented the family's diet with these "free" foods. In the May *quincena*, Delia, with her children, made nine excursions to the *milpa*
and the *monte*. She picked seven types of vegetables and greens,
three types of fruit, and, while washing clothes, caught shrimp and
eels. In July she had severe abdominal pains. She made two trips to
the doctor and received a series of injections. The total medical
expenses were only $4.60. This acute illness, however, significantly
changed her food procurement patterns. She did not have enough
energy, she said, to wash her clothes, make tortillas, or pick coffee,
let alone to go to the *milpa* or the *monte* to collect food. She also
did not make a trip to get free powdered milk from the church. In
all, she made just one excursion, to pick some *chipilin*. In October,
feeling well again, and in spite of a heavy work schedule (as shown
by her earnings of $26 a *quincena*), she gathered four types of
vegetables and greens and three types of fruit. In addition, she
bought more meat and fish (see Table 4.3).

DISCUSSION

These three case studies illustrate the interplay of several factors
influencing food procurement. The impact of health and illness on
the amount of time, energy, cash, and agricultural resources available for food provisioning is emphasized. These families illustrate
different illness situations and differential uses of various food-procuring strategies. They also show the impact of seasonality of food
crops and wage labor and the influence of household organization.

Health and Illness

Case A, Elena, had multiple problems. At a time that her own physical capacity was reduced, she had to devote more time and energy

to the care of ill household members. She compensated physically by cutting down on her own food-procuring activities. Elena's cash resources were low from June to mid August because of the "lean" work season, combined with continually increasing medical expenditures and debts.

Elena and her husband coped by selling corn from their *milpa*, when available, and by borrowing money from the *finquero*. During this period, the household food inventory was reduced to mainly corn and locally gathered greens, with hardly any consumption of meat and beans. This inadequate food inventory has a potentially synergistic effect in further increasing the vulnerability of household members to illness and thus decreasing their ability to function optimally.

The problems of a woman's ill health because of gynecological disorders, and excessive alcohol consumption by her husband, are illustrated in Case B, Teresa. This combination resulted in severely reduced cash income. Teresa resorted to extensive borrowing and buying on credit, spreading out her debts as much as possible, selling a pig to obtain cash, and increasing consumption of greens to augment the household food supply.

Case C, Delia, shows how an acute illness, such as gastritis, can profoundly disturb food procurement patterns. She reduced her energy expenditure by curtailing such household activities as washing clothes and critically reduced her gathering of wild foods, including greens, because of her illness. While greens are not a major energy source, they contribute to a better amino acid pattern and hence to the protein quality of the total diet. They are also a significant source of vitamin A activity, ascorbic acid, and iron.

Both Elena and Teresa use sequential or multiple treatment resources, which is characteristic of the health care strategies practiced by the finca population (Cosminsky and Scrimshaw 1980). Treating illness can result in medical debts and high cash expenditures, as in these case studies. Money that could have been allocated to procuring food may be spent on treatment and medicines instead. On the other hand, the need for food and a lack of cash may result in the avoidance or delay of medical care, thus prolonging and increasing the severity of the illness. Therefore, the interaction between illness, its treatment costs, and the household food supply may result in less than adequate food, spiraling debts, and suboptimal family nutritional status.

Seasonality

The critical periods for finca families are the peak season, when corn and cash are most plentiful, and the lean season, when they are scarce. The availability of human, agricultural, and cash resources, and the woman's use of options and strategies, differ in each of these seasons.

Peak Season.   The coffee harvest is from August to January, peaking from mid September through October. The main corn harvest is in August, with a second harvest in January. Corn is plentiful from mid August to April, so more cash is available for other items, including food, in contrast to the lean months, when corn must be purchased. The time and energy demands, however, are great for all family members, particularly the mother. Her hours of wage labor are increased. She must arise at three or four in the morning to prepare tortillas for breakfast and lunch and to wash the clothes before leaving to pick coffee.

Families can double their wages during the peak coffee season. For example, during the *quincena* October 14–28, Elena (Case A), together with her children, earned $20.00 and her husband earned $37.26; in July, the only income was around $17.00 a *quincena*, $11.00 of which went to buy corn. Similarly, Teresa (Case B), with her son Ruben, earned $41.60. The case also demonstrates how a woman, without help from her husband, but in favorable circumstances such as peak season and with help from her children, can bring the household back to food stability after a crisis.

Most women are eager to work during this period. They look forward to having more cash to spend as they wish. Women purchase more food, most of the yearly clothes and household articles, and pay off their debts. They buy more convenience foods, such as Protemas, pastas, and powdered soups, and high-protein foods, especially those preferred for lunches such as eggs, cheese, and meat (see Tables 4.2 and 4.3). There is also increased consumption of such valued foods as white sugar. Men use their extra income for food, to pay off some household debts and their personal debts for such items as radios or bicycles, and for alcohol. There is much variation among families in the household head's contribution to providing food during this period.

Lean Season.   During the slack period, from approximately April to August, the situation is drastically different because of shortages of corn and cash. The women now have more time and greater need for the procurement strategies described earlier in this chapter. For example, they gather more greens, which are regarded by some as poor men's food or for women and children, but are a critical item in times of food scarcity. This is also the season for fishing in the Salama River or in small streams. In addition, entrepreneurial activities may be extended by increased marketing projects or by more time spent on animal husbandry. Women may sell animals or their products, *panela*, or corn to obtain cash, as shown in the cases of Elena and Teresa.

With less cash available, a woman may have to buy on credit on the finca rather than at more favorable prices in outside markets and stores and may thus incur extensive debts. She may also borrow from neighbors, the finca owner, or other fincas and pay back the loan by picking coffee during the peak season. Elena and her husband both borrowed money in the lean months, committing themselves to paying it off by work in the peak season.

There is usually more sickness, especially children's diarrheal diseases, during this period (Valverde 1985). Women have more time to seek treatment and give family health care, but they usually do not have cash and frequently go into debt for this purpose.

It is during this lean period that the dependability of the husband's cash contribution to the family budget is particularly important. If he has to buy corn, he has little cash left to contribute to the rest of the food supply. If he keeps the remainder for his own spending, the family may be left short of necessities.

Household Organization

The household context significantly influences food procurement and health. Household composition (the size and age makeup of each household unit), the type of household (nuclear or extended), and the stage in the domestic cycle also affect women's responsibilities and duties or, conversely, the support they receive. Relations with members of other households in terms of support given or assistance requested depends primarily on the existence of kin, affinal, or fictive kin (godparent) relationships. Otherwise there is little cooperation and exchange between households.

A young nuclear family with several small children and no adolescent or older wage earners may depend on one income through most of the year. The mother is also constrained by the number of small children that she must care for alone, thus decreasing her mobility. These families have a high dependency ratio, resulting in what has been termed "dependency stress" by Marchione (1980). Not having as many options, they are more affected by the lean season. In this type of household the woman may resort to such low cash input strategies as finding and gathering greens, as illustrated in the cases of Elena and Delia.

In the "middle cycle family," which has both young and adolescent children, the older children help perform household duties (fetch water, prepare meals, take corn to the mill), are child caretakers, and serve as vendors for home-produced food items. They provide some income by working with the mother; by child caretaking, which frees the mother to work outside the home (on or off the finca); or by working independently on other fincas.

The mature (or older stage) household, which has adolescents, more adults, and few if any young children, may have a higher cash income per capita. The woman is free from reproductive activities and has control of enough cash of her own and her children's to engage in various entrepreneurial activities, such as running stores.

In both the middle and older households, women have the help of other adult women or older children—more human resources—as well as greater material resources (a sewing machine or a refrigerator, for example) that have been accumulated over time. These latter facilitate engaging in higher cash return enterprises, such as small stores.[6] They provide income that compensates for slack times and spreads out resources through the year.

In young nuclear families, or in other households where there is no child caretaker, women can seek work only seasonally at Finca San Felipe. In older households, some of the adult women work in outside plantations (where it is impossible to bring small children), and thus they can secure work throughout the year.

CONCLUSIONS

This chapter has examined the impact of the health status of women and their families on women's role as food provisioners and has focused on the microsocial and economic environments of the domestic unit in which women are embedded. This focus on the household has brought out the importance of the interrelationships between household members as they work together as a production and consumption unit and of the interrelationships between relatives in different households.

In subsistence agriculture the whole family cooperates in planting, maintaining, and harvesting their *milpa*. In the cash economy all adolescent and adult family members are expected to work for at least a portion of the year for cash wages on the finca. They are also expected to give the major portion of this income to the female household head for the family food supply. However, the proportion given varies widely among households and the gap between expectation and reality can be great.

The cash contribution of the men is often undependable because of alcohol consumption. This occurs most frequently on payday and results in direct loss of cash as well as loss of work days. Another factor that may seriously reduce the cash available for food is the amount that is spent for health care. A substantial proportion of the money a woman receives may be spent for medicines and treatment of household members. This variable reduction in cash

results in economic uncertainty and stress. At such times it is usually the woman who must manipulate available funds to best advantage and, in addition, attempt to extend her resource base to meet
the extra need.

The amount of cash and resources a woman is able to control
or amass is related to the seasons, to her own life cycle, and to her
place in the developmental cycle of the domestic group. Mature
women have more economic opportunities and more help from
family members; therefore, they can use a greater variety of strategies. Conversely, when a woman has many small children, she is
less likely to be able to take advantage of options.

The biological and health status of a woman is important in
her ability to function adequately. The reproductive stress of pregnancy and lactation are compounded by the nutritional stress of an
inadequate diet and by frequent infections. The resulting poor
health may limit a woman's ability to deal with everyday domestic
and provisioning activities and lowers her capacity to extend her
use of strategies and to cope with seasonal and household crises.

NOTES

Acknowledgments: Support for this study was provided by the International
Nutrition Program, Department of Nutrition and Food Science, Massa-
chusetts Institute of Technology, and Rutgers University Research Council
grants. The authors wish to express their appreciation to the owner and the
people of Finca San Felipe for their hospitality and kindness and to Nevin
Scrimshaw for his suggestions.

1. A "finca" can be defined as a tract of land used for agriculture or cattle
or both under a capitalistic system and employing one or more permanent
or temporary workers, who usually live on it with their families. A finca
may be owned by an individual, a family, a company, or the state. Approximately one-third of the population of Guatemala lives on plantations; living conditions there are among the worst for any group in the country
(Guatemala–A.I.D. 1977).

2. "Ladino" refers to people of Spanish or European culture and includes those who may be genetically Amerindian but who do not identify
themselves as Amerindian culturally.

3. In the study year the Guatemalan quetzal (Q) was par with the U.S. dollar ($).

4. These greens include *chipilin* (*Crotalaria longirostrata*), *hierba mora* (*Solanum nigrum* and *Solanum americanum*), *kishtan* (*Solanum wendlandii*), *berro* (watercress), *bledo* (wild amaranth), and squash leaves.

5. Pseudonyms are used in the case studies.

6. Six women, aged thirty-five to fifty-nine, earned from $700 to $2,960 a year, primarily from various entrepreneurial activities, such as midwifery or operating stores (Cosminsky and Scrimshaw 1981).

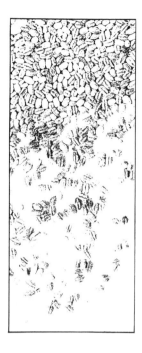

CHAPTER 5

Socioeconomic and Cultural Factors Affecting Interhousehold and Intrahousehold Food Distribution in Rural and Urban Bangladesh

Najma Rizvi

The aim of Najma Rizvi's research was to study patterns of food use as a basis for evaluating food and nutrition policy in Bangladesh by looking both at overall differences in diet between households and at differences in distribution within households. She initially made a distinction between environmental (or ecological) and cultural factors, one widely used in theory and practice in nutritional anthropology, and with a long tradition in anthropology generally. Trying to understand how and why different factors affected dietary practices led her not only to stress the significance of economic factors but also to present material that suggests the importance of relationships of inequality. Her research combines analysis of the interrelations between standard of living, diet, and domestic organization at a particular time with consideration of a system of social stratification. It also shows how the impact of cultural ideologies on the diets of domestic units and their members depends to a considerable extent on their place in such a system.

The households for which Rizvi collected data were selected to represent those with low, medium, and high incomes from rural and urban Bangladesh. This in itself makes her chapter both important and exceptional. Most ethnographic studies of dietary practices focus on a single income category (usually low) in either a rural or an urban area. Her selection of households made it possible for her to analyze the effects of major differences in incomes, and her material demonstrates some of the ways in which the activities and dietary practices of rich and poor households are interrelated.

Her analysis shows the inadequacy of the formulation of food and nutrition improvement strategies carried out by governmental and nongovernmental organizations. She advocates the involvement of anthropologists in policy formulation and implementation and the carrying out of more action research.

The purpose of the research on which this chapter is based, carried out during 1976 and 1977, was to study the complexity of factors affecting food use patterns in Bangladesh (Rizvi 1979). Households were selected as the basic units of study because in Bangladesh they are the primary consumption and budgeting units. It is also at this level that one can see most clearly how people use cultural "blueprints" to adapt to their specific environments and how their adaptations involve dietary practices. Households with low, middle, and high incomes were studied in both rural and urban environments, migration from rural to urban areas being a widespread and important phenomenon in Bangladesh.

An understanding of the interrelationships between socioeconomic and cultural factors and their effects on inter- and intrahousehold distribution of food is essential for formulating and implementing food and nutrition policy. This chapter has important policy implications, particularly because it shows the faulty assumptions underlying food and nutrition improvement strategies in Bangladesh.

SOCIOECONOMIC SETTING

The rural and urban sites where the research was carried out, Baliadi village and Dhaka city, are located in the same geographical region of Bangladesh, Baliadi village being situated about thirty-five miles north of Dhaka, the capital of Bangladesh.

Baliadi Village

Bangladesh is a land of villages, and Baliadi is one among some 65,000. When the research was carried out, Baliadi had a population of 1,669 people, who lived in an area of 146 acres. This high population density is typical of many rural areas in Bangladesh. A house-to-house survey, conducted during the initial phase of the fieldwork, showed that 63.85 percent of the total population of Baliadi were completely landless; 17.54 percent were marginal landholders, having less than one acre; 14.76 percent had from one to five acres; and only 3.85 percent had more than five acres.

Cultivation and Food.   The cropland of Baliadi is used primarily for the production of rice. Out of 110 acres of cropland, 84 acres were devoted to the cultivation of rice at the time of the research. About six years before the research was carried out, IRRI (high yielding variety) rice was introduced, replacing the traditional multiple cropping in most parts of the village, resulting in a decline in pulse (lentil) production—a major source of protein for the poor.[1] The application of chemical fertilizers and insecticides has also reduced the fish supply in Baliadi and many other rural areas. Rice, fish, pulses, and vegetables are the main foods in a Bangali diet. A variety of both wild and cultivated greens and vegetables are also used.

The majority of people in Baliadi buy their food. Even the landholding households, which can depend on homegrown rice and lentils, have to buy other foods from the market. Vegetables are grown in the backyards of many of the households, but this does not supply the major portion of the vegetables consumed. The village market sells rice, lentils, fish, poultry, vegetables, milk, oil, *gur* (unrefined sugar), and seasonal fruits. Beef, mutton, and poultry can be bought in the daily and weekly markets of the neighboring town some two miles away.

Most people eat three meals a day, but only cook once or twice a day. The preparation of meals in any household is an elaborate ritual in which all Baliadi women take great care and interest. In low-income households breakfast usually consists of leftover rice from the previous night. In the *bhadralok* (elite) homes hot boiled rice is usually served for breakfast with some vegetables or *dal* (lentils). The afternoon meal, the major one for all, is always freshly prepared. It consists of boiled rice and one or more preparations of subsidiary dishes of fish, vegetables, or *dal*. In the low-income households all foods, including rice, are prepared only once or twice a day to save cooking fuel (firewood, dry twigs, leaves). In high-income elite homes rice for dinner may be freshly cooked, but usually no subsidiary food is cooked at night.

Settlement and Social Units.   There are significant and complex social divisions within the village, and it is unrealistic to regard Baliadi as a single, homogeneous unit. There are nine distinct areas of settlement in the village, which are known locally as *paras*. These *paras* are largely occupied by kin-based groups, whose male members are related through patrilineal and patrilateral ties. They are distinguished and ranked on the basis of ancestral occupation, landholding, educational status, and religion. There are also economic and occupational differences within *paras*, and most have both landless and landholding households. Village groupings based on economic status and occupation cut across the *para* divisions.

Subdivisions within *paras* are called *bari*, a term that refers to both a homestead and an extended family group. A family in Bangladesh always means an extended family. A homestead often consists of the eldest male and his wife, their married sons and their wives and children, and their unmarried sons and daughters. Although as a rule married daughters do not establish their residence in their paternal home, sometimes a married daughter might set up her home in her father's *bhita* (land on which houses are built) if her husband has no ancestral land. A widow or a divorced daughter may also be attached to her parental home.

A clear distinction is drawn in Bangladesh between a family, which is a kin unit, even if traditionally sharing a homestead, and a household, which is a residential and consumption unit. The word for household is *ghar* (room) or *sansar* (consumption unit); Both center on the *chula* (hearth). Whenever a new household is formed, a separate *chula* is built beside the new living quarters of the married couple to symbolize the formation of a new household. Households can be nuclear or extended.

Occupations and Division of Labor.   Those with land, at all income levels, often combine their farming with other activities. The *bhadralok* (elite) may hold clerical and other positions in the city and employ others to work their land. Most poor work as agricultural and day laborers (on construction sites, in market centers) and as vendors; a few work as masons. Some landless, who have their own plows and draft animals, do sharecropping, but most of them work as seasonal agricultural laborers. Those with nonfarming backgrounds work as day laborers and vendors or follow such traditional occupations as working for the family of the landlord (an absentee landlord for some generations) in the city.

In Baliadi the separation between men's and women's work is most pronounced in the areas of cooking and agricultural labor. Farming is a man's occupation. The members of an extended family cooperate in doing the farm work and then distribute the produce among themselves. They also cooperate in running small businesses, such as shops in the village market. Day laborers and the *bhadralok* work individually in other nonagricultural pursuits. Men are also considered primarily responsible for maintaining the household, although women may supplement household income. Children often make important contributions in low-income households. One eight-year-old girl provided a major portion of the cash needed for daily food shopping (rice not included) by selling dry leaves she collected.

Although Baliadi women do not generally work in the fields, their contribution to rice culture is immense. Women perform all tasks related to the processing of rice, including parboiling, drying, dehusking, and winnowing. Whether members of nuclear or extended households, the women of a family cooperate with each other in doing such work. Sometimes even a woman from the same *para* may give a hand, although she does not have a share in the produce. All women of both *bhadralok* and non-*bhadralok* status engage in rice processing, although well-to-do *bhadralok* housewives usually hire female labor for doing such heavy work as dehusking. Since no rice crop comes into landless homes, these women have little of their own rice-processing work to do (their only rice being that paid to their husbands in exchange for agricultural work) and so may sell their labor to the *bhadralok* households. Also, a few women work as part-time helpers in well-to-do homes, two work in the local health center, two are teachers, and a few make jute bags and hammocks for a handicraft center in the village. In addition to their contribution to farming and their work for wages, women are responsible for the preparation of meals, child care, and keeping the dwellings and the courtyards clean. Women also grow some vegetables in their backyards, and women and girls cooperate in preparing meals. Men almost never assist with cooking, although they may sometimes look after the children. Since no men live by themselves, they never have to prepare meals.

Dhaka City

Dhaka, the capital and the largest city in Bangladesh, is ethnically and linguistically more homogeneous than other cities of similar size in the Indian subcontinent. With the exception of a small minority of Hindus and Christians, all the inhabitants are Muslims, the great majority of whom speak Bangla. The Muslim Bangalis are differentiated by the distinction between *Dhakaiya* and non-*Dhakaiya* (those who retain no ties with the countryside and those who do) and by economic status. In the city there is a much greater variety in life-styles, and a more clearly marked difference between rich and poor, than there is in Baliadi. The neighborhoods are not primarily kin-based groups as they are in the village, although kin may live in close proximity. But the term "family" always means an extended group, and households, as in the village, can be nuclear or extended.

All urban households depend solely on the market for their food. The daily markets of the city offer many kinds of fresh produce. The amount and variety of fish, vegetables, and fruits are much greater than in the small rural markets. There are also meat and poultry and egg shops, small grocery stores, larger general stores, food peddlers, and many different kinds of restaurants and tea shops. Poor households, however, do not have the means to make use of these many sources of food.

The occupational structure of the city shows wide variation. Many new urban residents work as day laborers, which includes rickshaw driving, transporting goods, working on construction projects, and selling various types of goods. A few are office "peons" (messengers and caretakers), security guards, or taxi drivers. The educated elite men do white-collar jobs ranging from low-paid clerks to highly paid professionals.

A very small proportion of city women work outside the household. While in the village the work world of men and women is strictly segregated, this is not so in the city. In the elite, high-income group, women work as professors, doctors, engineers, architects, schoolteachers, and bank personnel. As a rule, women do not work as waitresses, salesclerks, shopkeepers, office caretakers, or in construction. Low-income working women most often are employed as full-time or part-time domestic help. In the city, the system of *purdah* (seclusion of women) persists, although to a lesser degree than in the village. Unlike the rural elite women, who observe *purdah* more than others, the city elite women observe it less than other women. And while the system of *purdah* does not restrict a poor village woman from moving around her neighborhood, the city women and young girls living in slums remain confined to their own immediate surroundings.

Cooking and child care are the primary responsibilities of women in all groups. But whereas in the village women in all socioeconomic groups participate themselves in these activities, elite city women usually have hired help and often play only a supervisory role in cooking and child care. In the middle-income group, some part-time help is available for doing the heavy tasks, but for the most part the adult women do their own cooking. In all groups the mother is assisted in taking care of the children either by her own older children, other family members, or hired domestic help. The fathers and adult male members occasionally help care for young children, but, as in the village, they do not generally help with the cooking.

DATA COLLECTION

The first stage was the selection of a rural site, within a reasonable distance of Dhaka, inhabited by people of different socioeconomic backgrounds. Having found Baliadi village, and selected households for study, urban households were chosen whose families had originally come from the district where Baliadi is located (or neighboring districts, where food habits were similar to those in Baliadi).

The Rural Sample

Following some participant observation and a survey of the village, twenty-five households were chosen, representing all socioeconomic groups and all eight Muslim *paras* in the village. The sample included households of various sizes, both nuclear and extended; in only one was there no father present. The largest household had twelve members and the smallest three. The households in the low-income group were relatively smaller and had a lower adult to child ratio than the other two groups.

   The number of landless in the sample was proportional to landless in the village, which was more than 60 percent. The primary occupation of this group was wage work of various types. Only three households in the sample depended primarily on their own farming for a livelihood; of these, two were sharecroppers and one farmed his own land. The majority of rural mothers did not work for wages. Of the twenty-five sample mothers, only four worked outside their own households: Two worked as helpers in the houses of the rural elite, one made jute goods, and the fourth taught in school. Thirteen of the sample households had low incomes, eight were in the middle-income category, and four had high incomes (Table 5.1). The educational status of the fathers and mothers varied with income, and the educational status of the

T A B L E   5.1
Number of Rural and Urban Households in Different Income Groups
(Per-Capita Monthly Income)

	Rural	Urban*
Low	Less than 50 takas 13	Less than 80 takas 20
Middle	50 90 takas 8	80 120 takas 4
High	Over 90 takas 4	Over 120 takas 8

*Because urban living entails greater expenses, a higher cutoff point has been used for the urban sample. $U.S. 1 = 15 takas.

mothers in each income group was as a whole lower than that of the fathers.

The Urban Sample

In locating households for the urban sample, help was sought from people of different backgrounds from both Baliadi and Dhaka. Thirty-two households (*Dhakaiya* and non-*Dhakaiya*) were selected with great variations in size and composition, income, education, and occupations. A pronounced difference was found between the monthly income of the richest (9,500 takas per month) and the poorest (20 takas per month) households, much greater than in the village. The household with the highest income was that of a factory owner; the one with the lowest income was headed by a widowed mother, who worked as a domestic in a neighboring well-to-do home. Only in this poorest home and in one other was no father present.

The proportion of mothers employed, although greater than in the rural sample, was nevertheless small. Three of them supplemented their income by selling foods prepared at home; their children were important in helping with this activity. Two of the mothers worked as domestics; one was an elementary-school teacher; and two with graduate degrees taught and did administrative work. The average size of the city households was slightly smaller than that of the rural households, and, as in the rural sample, the poor households were slightly smaller than those with higher incomes.

Methods of Data Collection

Participant observation and informal, unstructured interviewing were the main methods used in gathering information. No direct questions were asked about food distribution; Instead, the approach was to observe carefully behavior associated with food distribution and its relationship to other aspects of culture. Standardized interviewing procedures were used only to fill out forms on household consumer expenditures, food intake (frequency of intake), and children's feeding patterns.

Women (mothers and grandmothers) were the primary informants for the data relating to cooking, distribution of food, and feeding of children. Men provided data relating to food production and the buying of goods. Information on landholding was collected at the level of the household, and that on income, education, and occupation was recorded for individual members. The total incomes of working members were added to get the household income data, and the educational status of the household was determined by the highest level of education present. The frequency of consumption of foods and the consumer expenditure surveys were recorded at the household level.

Pregnancy and postpartum food beliefs and food use data were collected from individual adult females through meal and snacking patterns while they were going through these states, as well as by interacting with mothers and grandmothers. Data on the onset and duration of breast feeding and supplementary feeding (liquid and solid) were collected for the youngest child member of the household. No attempt was made to quantify the data on food beliefs, food categories, and values associated with the distribution of food. In order to achieve greater reliability, quantitative data collected through interviewing were always verified by participant observation. The use of various methods to elicit information helped in attaining greater precision in understanding the complexity of the factors affecting food behavior and nutrition.

FOOD, CULTURE, AND RELATIONSHIPS

Food classification in the study areas was found to be based on five categories: strength-giving foods, blood-producing foods, "hot" and "cold" foods, "nirdosh"/"nirog" (fault and disease free) foods, and bitter foods (the local medicines). Beliefs about food and social relationships involved gender roles; rules of hospitality; and the particular situations of pregnant, postpartum, and lactating women and of infants and young children. All these beliefs can, under certain circumstances, affect use and distribution of food within and between households and the nutrition of vulnerable categories of people (Rizvi 1979, 1986).

Rice

Rice is the staple food of Bangalis, rich and poor, educated and uneducated, rural and urban. Served boiled, it forms the major part of a meal, and it supplies 70–80 percent of the total calories consumed. In the Bangla language rice and food are synonymous—eating rice means having one's meal. Foods are classified into the "main food," rice, and the "side food," everything other than rice, except wheat products and sweet potatoes, which are considered "rice substitutes." In Bangladesh a distinction is made between a meal and a snack, based on the presence or absence of rice. The mere presence of rice in any form, however, does not constitute a meal. The rice has to be served boiled, or fried in oil or butter, for there to be a meal. Not all rice is equally valued. Parboiled rice (*shiddha*) is preferred to unparboiled (*atop*). People also tend to have a negative attitude to IRRI rice, which is considered to have a flat taste or none at all.

Given the central importance of rice in the diet of Bangalis, it is not surprising that wheat is not readily accepted as a substitute, even though it is cheaper. When day laborers receive wheat for their wages, they often will sell it and buy half the amount of rice. During the preharvest season or in the monsoon months, when poor people are underemployed, they are forced to eat wheat because it is cheaper than rice. But they always look forward to the rice harvesting season, when they can find farm work and bring home rice, and when they can also afford to buy rice because the prices go down.

Subsidiary Food Items

Rice is eaten with a variety of preparations of fish, vegetables, lentils, and occasionally meat. Although all big fish are considered nutritious, only the *jiol mach* are believed to have blood-producing properties. In the local categorization of food these fish also have a high prestige value and belong in the "nirdosh" or "nirog" categories of food. Although vegetables are not highly regarded, they are categorized as being balanced in their inherent characteristics, with the exception of radish, pumpkin, eggplant, and some varieties of *shag* (greens). Similarly, lentils are not highly valued but are widely eaten, and most of the many varieties recognized are considered "nirdosh" by all groups. Finally, although Bangalis in general, and rural Bangalis in particular, do not show great preference for meat, its occasional use is desired by all. In the meat group mutton and chicken are considered to be "nirdosh" and young chicken to be particularly nutritious. Beef and duck are considered "hot."

Food for Pregnancy and for Postpartum Women

Contrary to popular belief, the village women do recognize the increasing need for food in pregnancy. Also, they believe that by eating more less space will be available for the baby, which in turn will ensure an easy delivery. Pregnancy restrictions are rare in Bangladesh, and the foods that are restricted, such as big fish, do not generally appear in the poor household's food menu. Malnutrition in pregnancy cannot be ascribed to beliefs and lack of knowledge.

The postpartum period being considered a particularly vulnerable time, a broader set of dietary rules, both prescriptions and proscriptions, is present. The dietary rules are expected to help the mother to get back to a normal state of health and to prevent illness in the mother and the baby. The first six days after delivery are considered the most critical for both. At this time fish, meat, lentils, and greens are to be avoided to prevent gastrointestinal disorders. The late postpartum period is less restrictive, and at this time eating blood-producing fish with rice and other strength-giving foods is emphasized.

Solid Foods for Young Children

The young children between the ages of six months and two years face the highest risk of malnutrition because of inadequate intake. The general belief among mothers in Baliadi and Dhaka is that a child is not ready to eat any solids until some important biological signals begin to appear. Comparison of some of these signals with indicators described in the scientific literature shows that they are essentially similar (Rizvi 1979). But despite such similarities, interpretation of these signals in both Baliadi and Dhaka generally leads to delaying the introduction of solid foods beyond the age at which children should receive them. This in turn makes the children especially vulnerable to particular nutritional deficiencies after six months, or earlier in cases where mother's milk or supplementary feeding is inadequate, a situation most likely to arise in poor households. In contrast, in the United States disregarding of these signals by mothers and doctors can lead to too early introduction of solid foods and to different problems, such as the development of allergic reactions to some foods.

While the readiness of a child to eat solids depends on the appearance of some biological indications, the type of food a child may eat depends on the availability of various types of foods cooked in the home and on beliefs concerning foods suitable for young children. As the "superfood" and the food most readily available in all households, rice is the first food to be given to most children. But it is also believed that early eating of rice will produce a potbelly. Again, although most fish are considered neither "hot" nor "cold" and are not therefore associated with any negative properties, the same fish are believed to cause worms in children. Beef, being a "hot" food, is to be avoided by young children. Greens are not thought appropriate for them, because they provide only roughage. This is particularly considered to be the case when the child has diarrhea. Fears that various foods will cause gastrointestinal disorders (diarrhea, dysentery, worms) in young children are widespread and important, since both diarrhea and worms are serious health hazards and are endemic in Bangladesh.

Diarrhea, a "hot" illness, requires the avoidance of such "hot" foods as milk and also requires the eating of such "cool" foods as barley. Preventive measures for controlling children's diarrhea caused by natural (the breaking of postpartum taboos and so on) rather than supernatural (*kharab batash*—mysterious air—or the "evil eye") factors are following of food rules by the mother in the postpartum period and, again, delay in the giving of solids. Curative measures are the withdrawal of milk (though not breast milk) and of all solids from the children's diet, together with the use of both herbal and Western medicines. The inability of children below the age of two years to fend for themselves also limits their consumption of some foods, such as fruits. Older children in the village can wander around and satisfy part of their nutrient needs by gathering foodstuffs.

Gender

Other cultural beliefs relate not only to what food items should be eaten, at what times, and by what categories of people, but also to how food should be distributed within the household. All quality subsidiary foods, it is thought, should be apportioned by status, a particular distinction being made between men and women. In Bangladesh the adult male household members, particularly the head of the household, enjoy the highest status. This is articulated through a number of symbolic behaviors, which begin soon after the birth of the child—for example, the custom of doing *azan* (the call for prayer) at the birth of a boy but not at the birth of a girl. But although symbolically the higher status of male children is articulated early, all children grow up in a highly permissive environment up to the age of four or five. Although in some urban elite homes attention is paid to discipline at an early age, in most households a young child is rarely spanked. On the contrary, parents and other members of the household try to meet the children's demands whenever possible.

At the age of five or six, however, girls begin to help their mothers with domestic tasks in all but urban elite homes. Boys start with only a few small tasks at that age, but by eight or ten they are shopping, assisting with other chores, and sometimes helping their fathers. After the age of eleven or twelve the sexual division of labor is complete. From this age on in Baliadi the girls are no longer allowed to wander around the village, their movements being confined to their own *bari* (homestead) or to the *para* (neighborhood). *Purdah* (seclusion of young girls and women from men) is practiced by all in the village, but the degree varies with differences in socioeconomic status, the elite village women remaining more secluded than the nonelite.

It is also believed that among young children boys should not be given preference over girls in the distribution of subsidiary foods, but again even in the early years some distinctions are made between the sexes. Thus, for example, while it is thought to be all right for a boy to demand additional servings of such quality foods as fish, a girl's demand for more of the same is considered a sign of *alakhi* (bad luck). From the age of six or seven, when the indulging period is over, it is considered appropriate for boys to be given priority over girls; the latter are taught correspondingly how to behave, learning the value of patience and that it is not appropriate to demand a larger share of anything. For example, when a six-year-old girl asked for a second serving of fish, her mother complied with the request, but at the same time emphasized that girls should learn to eat their share of rice with a small amount of fish. Her mother said, "It is right for you to eat this way in your parents' home, but what would you do when you go to your husband's?" From an early age girls are taught that an ideal woman is one who is satisfied with little and is capable of any kind of self-sacrifice.

Hospitality

Finally, hospitality rules also specify how food should be shared and distributed. In both the Bangali and Muslim traditions food is regarded as an important medium for showing warmth, so that guests should be served food. Whether a guest should receive a full meal, a snack, tea, or *pan* (betel leaves) depends on the status of the guest in relation to the household members. In even the poorest households women will go to great lengths to serve their guests appropriate foods. This may be particularly difficult where, as can often happen, guests come unannounced. Where there are limited supplies of food, the rules of hospitality, combined with the highly valued quality of self-sacrifice in women, leads them to forego their share of the subsidiary foods. If the guest is a woman, she eats with other female members of the household, but she is always given a larger share of the subsidiary foods than they are.

INTER- AND INTRAHOUSEHOLD VARIATION IN PATTERNS OF FOOD CONSUMPTION

The cultural values and beliefs related to food are to some extent held by all members of both the rural and urban samples, although modified in some respects by members of the educated urban elite (Rizvi 1979). The differences between households seem to lie particularly in the frequency with which they are expressed and the extent to which they are acted on. The villagers and poor urbanites with little formal education seem to express the traditional beliefs more often than middle- and upper-income educated people in the city, possibly because of the particular relevance of these beliefs to their lives. Thus, for example, the rural and urban poor, who live under continuous threat of various types of infections, believe in the medicinal value of bitter foods more strongly than the educated middle- and upper-income urbanites. In addition, poor postpartum women who are unable to eat recommended foods, which are expensive, observe restrictions more carefully than do elite women who can follow the recommended diets. Considerable variation in the extent to which preferences, prescriptions, and restrictions were followed within the rural and the urban sample can be related to the social and economic circumstances of households and to variations in domestic organization.

The Household Level

Differences in food consumption were calculated with two measures: (1) the frequency of use of rice, fish, meat, *dal* (lentils), *shag* (greens), and other foods (Table 5.2); and (2) the dietary complexity score, which was calculated by adding the frequency score of items used in the household. In both the rural and urban sample, there was considerable variation between households in the use of subsidiary food items, but there was a marked similarity in the frequency of consumption of rice. There was also more frequent consumption of fish than meat in both samples, although urban households ate meat more often than the rural ones. The range of

TABLE 5.2
Frequency of Use of Various Foods

	Rural (N = 25)					Urban (N = 31)				
	Seldom	2 Times a Week	4 Times a Week	7 Times a Week	14 Times a Week	Seldom	2 Times a Week	4 Times a Week	7 Times a Week	14 Times a Week
Rice					25 (100%)					31 (100%)
Wheat	17 (68%)		1 (4%)	6 (24%)	1 (4%)	13 (42%)	3 (10%)		15 (49%)	
Fish	1 (4%)	13 (52%)	7 (28%)	3 (12%)	1 (4%)	2 (6%)	12 (39%)	7 (23%)	5 (16%)	5 (16%)
Beef	25 (100%)					24 (77%)	4 (13%)	1 (3%)	2 (6%)	
Chicken	25 (100%)					25 (81%)	2 (6%)	2 (6%)	1 (3%)	1 (3%)
Mutton	25 (100%)					26 (84%)	2 (6%)	1 (3%)		2 (6%)
Eggs	21 (84%)	3 (12%)		1 (4%)		24 (77%)	1 (3%)	1 (3%)	5 (16%)	
Milk	13 (52%)	6 (24%)		5 (20%)	1 (4%)	23 (74%)	2 (6%)	1 (3%)	4 (13%)	1 (3%)
Dal	2 (8%)	11 (44%)	11 (44%)	1 (4%)			20 (65%)	1 (3%)	3 (10%)	7 (23%)
Vegetables		11 (44%)		13 (52%)	1 (4%)		2 (6%)	1 (3%)	13 (42%)	15 (48%)
Shag			18 (72%)	7 (28%)		3 (10%)	24 (77%)	3 (10%)	1 (3%)	

Note: Percentages may not add to exactly 100 because of rounding.

variation between households in the use of subsidiary foods was highest for fish and meats and lowest for vegetables. Given the great similarity in frequency of consumption of rice, differences in dietary complexity resulted from variation in the consumption of other food items. What factors, then, can be seen as leading to similarities and differences in consumption at the household level?

People in all economic positions, whether rural or urban, believe that rice is a "superfood," and that belief is manifest in its generally high frequency of use. Nevertheless, the type of rice consumed can be seen to be related to household income and purchasing power. Thus, in the rural areas rich farmers make a profit growing IRRI rice, which enables them to buy traditional varieties of rice for their own use, varieties that are considered to be better tasting and that are always sold at a higher price. Poor rural and urban households are forced to buy IRRI and *atop* (unparboiled rice) because it is the cheapest available, despite the prevalent belief that such rice has no food value.

Variation in the use of subsidiary food items also cannot be explained by food beliefs alone. Despite the view that vegetables and *dal* have no important food value, they are eaten more frequently than fish, which is perceived to be of high food value. The relation between the eating of these foods (as shown in the measure of dietary complexity and frequency of food use) and various features of the sample households was examined to try to explain the variation in consumption of subsidiary food items. The characteristics of the households considered were income, education, occupation, rural or urban residence, number of working adults, size of household, and structure and type of household.

The relationship of each of the variables to dietary complexity and frequency of use of different foods could be analyzed by either qualitative or quantitative means. In examining these relationships both approaches were employed. The quantitative analysis was carried out using a regression model. In doing the statistical analysis the two samples were combined because of small sample size. For this reason, landholding status could not be included as a variable. The effect of landholding status, however, was incorporated into cash income by calculating the price of agricultural output and then adding it to cash income, and qualitative material was also used in analyzing its effects.

In the regression analysis, the most powerful single predictor of dietary complexity is income, and the combined effect of income and education (themselves highly correlated) reaches a value of .914. The effect of urban location is not as strong as income and education. Although it is true that there are more foods available in Dacca, urbanization in itself does not lead to diversity in the diet of all city dwellers. Only those with high incomes are able to benefit from the variety of foods in the city.

No relationship was found between the number of working members in the household and dietary complexity in the sample as a whole. However, such a relationship was evident in the high-income group. The presence of additional working members in the low-income group does not necessarily lead to greater complexity in the diet, because the increase in income from the presence of an additional working member is too small to make any appreciable difference to the quality of the diet. In the low-income households, which are more often nuclear than extended, the children work from a very young age to supplement income.

When the R value was calculated for fish, beef, mutton, chicken, eggs, milk, *dal*, vegetables, and greens separately, income came out to be the most important single predictor of the frequency of consumption of eggs, beef, mutton, and *dal*, and the second most important predictor in the case of milk, fish, and chicken. Income and education together explained more than 70 percent of the frequency variation in fish, chicken, mutton, eggs, milk, and *dal*. Urban location and income showed a greater relationship than income and education in the use of beef and mutton. This is in agreement with the general observation that the use of meat was more frequent in the urban than in the rural sample, probably because of greater availability.

Households with landholdings of more than one acre were found to be at a particular advantage in the consumption of fish, milk, and eggs because they owned cows, chickens, and ponds for raising fish. Neither income nor landholding status appears to have any direct effect on the frequency of use of vegetables and greens.

But the kinds of greens used and their sources are different in different households. The two varieties of *shag* (*pat*—jute greens and *kaloi*—lentil greens) that are most preferred by landless and landholding alike are usually consumed only by landholding households, which can grow them. They are not sold in the village market, and those who gather them from other people's fields risk insult and abuse. Women and children from low-income households more often gather wild greens that grow around the edges of rice fields and in other open areas.

The overriding importance of economic status for food consumption and dietary quality can also be seen by analyzing the household expenditure patterns of different income groups. There is no question of low-income households budgeting their resources unwisely: They have too few resources. Low-income households spend a much higher proportion of their funds on food, and on individual food items, than high-income groups, even though their diets show less dietary complexity (see Table 5.3). The low-income urban households appear to be in a better position in this respect than their rural counterparts, but this is probably not the case, since they have to pay rent and higher prices for all consumer goods and also have no possibility of collecting food.

Intrahousehold Food Distribution

Distribution of food within the household is important in determining the food consumption and dietary quality of household members. Beliefs and values outlined earlier relating to the differential status of men and women, hospitality, pregnancy and postpartum periods, and the care and feeding of young children might be expected to affect intrahousehold distribution. This is the case, but the way in which, and the extent to which, they affect distribution depend on the combined effect of people's economic circumstances and the nature of the households in which they live.

In none of the sample households was the available food distributed equally among all members. Unequal distribution of rice could be explained by age differences, but such was not the case for unequal distribution of other foods, especially animal proteins.

T A B L E 5.3

Average Monthly Expenditure and Percentage of Income Spent on Food and Cooking Fuel

	Low Income (N = 13) (Average Income—200.83 takas)		High Income (N = 4) (Average Income—1,550 takas)	
	Average Monthly Expenses (Takas)	Percentage	Average Monthly Expenses (Takas)	Percentage
Rural				
Food				
Rice	138.50	68.96	453.75	29.27
Fish	11.33	5.64	35.00	2.25
Vegetables	12.58	6.26	31.25	2.01
Meat	—	—	20.00	1.29
Dal	5.75	2.86	8.75	0.56
Milk	5.23	2.60	37.50	2.41
Eggs	0.46	0.22	3.00	0.19
Spices	18.33	9.12	27.25	1.75
Oil	7.58	3.77	19.75	1.27
TOTAL (food only)	199.76	99.43	636.25	41.00
Cooking fuel	22.08	10.99	42.50	2.74
TOTAL (food and fuel)	221.84	110.42	678.75	43.74

	Low Income (N = 19)* (Average Income—330.21 takas)		High Income (N = 8) (Average Income—2,887.5 takas)	
	Average Monthly Expenses (Takas)	Percentage	Average Monthly Expenses (Takas)	Percentage
Urban				
Food				
Rice	157.42	47.67	385.00	13.33
Fish	25.00	7.59	215.00	7.44
Vegetables	22.74	6.89	122.80	4.25
Meat	3.00	0.90	186.87	6.47
Dal	10.42	3.16	21.87	0.75
Milk	7.47	2.26	123.75	4.29
Eggs	2.78	0.84	91.75	3.17
Spices	15.78	4.78	63.25	2.19
Oil	13.11	3.98	72.37	2.50
TOTAL (food only)	257.72	78.07	1282.66	44.39
Cooking fuel	32.63	9.88	53.62	1.85
TOTAL (food and fuel)	290.35	87.95	1336.28	46.24

*Information was not available for the twentieth household.

The effect of household size, composition, and type were examined in an attempt to understand the differences in patterns of distribution observed. Household size as such did not seem to affect food distribution; it became important only when viewed in relation to income. Large households with low income and with a higher ratio of children to adults did allocate a smaller share of subsidiary foods to women and children. Neither size nor composition had a marked effect on the distribution of food in high-income households, since there was plenty of food for everyone.

Similarly, patterns of distribution that favored men over women and placed a high priority on hospitality only led to detrimental inequalities in consumption of food in households where there were inadequate resources and insufficient food to meet the needs of the whole household. Even in low-income households, mothers in charge of the distribution of food did not distinguish between male and female children below about five or six years. But the disparity between the girls' and the boys' share of quality food increased with age and reached a maximum when women became mothers. In the low-income households it was found that the cooked weight of a child's share of fish curry ranged from 15 to 30 grams, the mother's share from 0 to 45 grams, and the father's share from 38 to 128 grams. In the high-income, educated households of the city, a child's share varied from 40 to 100 grams, the mother's from 40 to 250 grams, and the father's from 65 to 350 grams. In low-income extended households, where a mother-in-law was in charge of distribution, the young mother often received a larger share of subsidiary foods. Where the young mother herself controlled distribution, she usually served herself last and so often had an even smaller share of the limited subsidiary food.

Furthermore, in poor homes when visitors were present, the mother and other adult female members of the household received even smaller portions than usual, since they had no money to buy more food for their visitors but gave instead what they would usually eat themselves. Even in high-income households, eating arrangements sometimes affected distribution of food. In upper-income rural households, where women ate after men, women might on occasion be left with lesser amounts of food. In contrast, in urban high-income households, where male and female members more often ate together, this was less likely.

Inequality in the distribution of food to women and children was further affected by various food beliefs and taboos relating to the postpartum period; pregnancy restrictions, being few, did not have much effect. As already described, lack of awareness of the increasing food needs of children and delay in the introduction of solid foods are important factors affecting distribution of food to young children. Concerns about indigestion and diarrhea and the beliefs associated with prevention and cure of gastrointestinal disorders further reduce the children's intake. But again, because of the patterns of disease characteristic of households of different economic status, and because of the way in which income affects the observation of dietary prescriptions and prohibitions, beliefs about food tend to have a greater detrimental effect on dietary quality of young children of low-income households. Another reason members of such households observe dietary prohibitions more strictly is their inability to afford foods that are recommended and prescribed for certain physical states, such as postpartum and lactation, and for good health in general. Since they are unable to eat foods that will make them strong and healthy, they believe that they are more at risk of suffering from ill health if they fail to observe taboos and restrictions (Rizvi 1979).

CONCLUSION

The research presented in this paper shows that household food use patterns were the outcome of a complex interrelationship between cultural and socioeconomic factors at all income levels in both rural and urban areas. It also shows that, contrary to the assumptions underlying nutrition intervention programs in Bangladesh, malnutrition resulted primarily from economic deprivation and only secondarily from cultural and social factors. The structure and organization of households, and beliefs relating to the distribution of food within households, did not in themselves lead to malnutrition.

The two main strategies for nutrition improvement that were used in Bangladesh were both based on the general assumption that the poor suffering from malnutrition were ignorant of good nutritional practices. The first, nutrition education programs, used oral and written materials to teach the importance of maintaining good health, the nutritive properties of different foods, good budgeting practices, and the value of cleanliness. The second, feeding programs, which theoretically recognized the importance of poverty as well as ignorance, distributed milk powder, baby food in jars, and "high protein" cookies. Both approaches were based on faulty assumptions.

Contrary to the premise of the nutrition education programs, a high priority is placed on good health, particularly the health of children, in poor nonliterate households. Nonliterate rural and urban people have no knowledge of the nutrient composition of foods, but the local categorization of foods (into strength- and energy-giving foods and blood-producing foods) shows that they are also aware of the relationship between the eating of certain foods and the maintenance of good health. The foods categorized as blood producing and strength giving happen to include those rich in protein. The beneficial effect of prolonged breast feeding is recognized by all, but poor women, who tend to breast feed their children longer, are frequently malnourished and often complain about producing less milk.

Poor households make good use of what resources they have, and the "low cost" nutritious meals recommended by nutrition educators were often more expensive than any poor household could afford. In encouraging women to feed their children more *dal, shag*, and fish, those carrying out the nutrition education programs also undermined the women by criticizing them, instead of recognizing the very real limitations on what they could obtain and the reality of the severity of diarrheal disease and worm infestation. Finally, the education programs recommended cleanliness without providing people with the means to clean themselves, including the money to purchase soap, and ensuring a clean water supply.

The advocates of feeding programs argued that any food given to the poor would improve nutrition. They said that the magnitude of the problem of malnutrition demanded immediate action and, consequently, that the occasional distribution of milk powder, milk–wheat gruel, high-protein cookies, and jars of baby food would be beneficial. These feeding programs may have succeeded in saving a few lives from starvation, but they did not improve the nutrition of mothers and children. On the contrary, they undermined the confidence of mothers in the nutritive value of breast milk and also led them to believe that foods showing pictures of healthy babies might have a magical effect on their children's health. What nutrition education there was in these programs also emphasized cultural factors rather than the role of poverty.

On the basis of the knowledge gained doing this research, in 1979 I presented an alternative program for nutrition improvement that attempted to meet some of the inadequacies of the then existing nutrition improvement programs (Rizvi 1979). The suggested program included both research and action components dealing with improvement in economic status and the health environment and with nutrition education. In view of the particular need of nutritional improvement for mothers and children, the action research was designed to focus on this group, although the benefits were not to be limited to them. The hypotheses to be tested included

1. Improving nutrition of the mother–child dyad requires an improvement in the economic status of the household. Any separate attempt to better the nutrition of this vulnerable group without enhancing the general economic status of the household is likely to be a failure
2. Nutrition education without improvement of economic status will be mostly ineffective
3. Nutrition education stressing the importance of giving solid foods will achieve some success if the incidence of diarrhea and worm infestation is reduced

In August 1980, as part of the Second Five-Year Plan, a food policy known as the Food Security Plan was introduced in Bangladesh (Rizvi 1983). Its main goal was to ensure a minimum level of consumption, chiefly by an increase in cereal production. It also involved procuring food at a price that gave incentives to farmers and an open market sale of rice and wheat during lean periods to reduce high prices. Other strategies designed to help feed the poor included modified rationing, available to rural households only; distributing relief foods to the disadvantaged; and food for work.

For reasons discussed in more detail elsewhere (Rizvi 1983) the strategies followed under the Food Security Plan did not have the desired results. Although there were some problems in the implementation and administration of the plan, the major reason for its lack of effectiveness was that it did not deal with the main causes of malnutrition among the poor in Bangladesh. Although those who formulated the Food Security Plan were aware of inequalities in income and distribution of land, and of the particularly vulnerable position of women and children, they did not take these factors into account in devising courses of action.

The research presented here has shown that if the economic status of poor households is not improved, together with the health environment, and particular attention is not paid to the situation of women and young children, it is unlikely that the severity of malnutrition will be reduced substantially. It also suggests that anthropologists have an important contribution to make to the formulation of food and nutrition policy, and that the collaborative input of economists, anthropologists, and nutritionists is needed to create an effective policy.

NOTE

1. Increase in the cultivation and use of wheat in Bangladesh as a whole is discussed in Lindenbaum 1986.

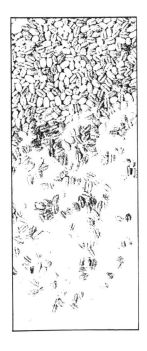

CHAPTER 6

Kin Ties, Food, and Remittances in a Garifuna Village in Southern Belize

Joseph Palacio

*Joseph Palacio starts from the British anthropological tradition of
the study of food and social relations. He sees his orientation as
related to Firth's ([1936] 1957) "alimentary approach" to kinship,
and he uses Nadel's (1956) concept of role. But he also draws on
cultural and cognitive anthropology, and studies of economic development, to produce a flexible analysis of a situation that illustrates some of the profound changes that have taken place in
many of the societies traditionally studied by anthropologists. No
other studies of dietary practices have been carried out in this kind
of situation, and his analysis presents new material and new ways
of looking at it.*

*His research was conducted in Lisurnia (pseudonym), a Gar-
ifuna village in southern Belize. The site was isolated, marginal,
and neglected by government, and there had been general migration of able-bodied men and women in search of work to towns
and cities in Belize and to the United States. Young children, however, frequently remained behind, cared for by grandparents and
others through the Garifuna system of fosterage. Their care was
paid for by remittances from the migrants. Since the villagers produced little of their own food supply, remittances for food purchases were essential for the survival of many households.*

*Thus Palacio's study shows a situation where households de-
pend on a geographically widespread network of relationships for
basic necessities, including food. His detailed analysis of fosterage
also demonstrates great flexibility in a cultural system where continuity in values and definitions of relationships is associated with
marked changes in the actual composition, organization, and dietary practices of domestic units. His presentation of case studies
of domestic units shows the parts played by men, women, and children in obtaining, allocating, and using food and other resources; the conflicts and problems that arise; the interventions of
villagers; and the resulting diet and health of the members of
households. Given the adverse economic conditions, he questions
the possibility of such villages as Lisurnia surviving without the
provision of new local employment opportunities for some of
those who otherwise have to migrate to find work.*

W ithin the last thirty years influences from outside the Circum-Caribbean area have had far-reaching effects on Garifuna rural communities in Belize and elsewhere, particularly as a result of outmigration and increasing reliance on a cash economy. The outmigration of the working population has left some villages inhabited primarily by children under fourteen and adults over fifty. Reliance on a cash economy has been associated with a decline in subsistence food production and dependence on the purchase of food for survival. The process of marginalization has resulted in whole villages becoming, in effect, dependent on relationships with close kin working in cities.

Such early anthropological studies as those of Firth ([1936] 1957), who first used the "alimentary approach" to kinship, showed how the analysis of food-related behavior could lead to an understanding of the maintenance of kin ties and of the ways in which the norms and relationships of kinship define how food is acquired and used. These early studies were carried out in small communities, where it was relatively easy to observe a wide range of behavior. The research on which this chapter is based shows the importance of kin relationships built around exchange of material items (food and other necessities) for the widely dispersed Garifuna, who are located partly in coastal villages in northeastern Central America, partly in cities and towns in their respective countries, and partly in the United States.

The study focuses on the process of food acquisition as the main aspect of food behavior. It argues that cash remittances, which enter the household as a part of fosterage relationships, are a major means of acquiring food. It demonstrates the relationship between receipt of remittances and certain conditions within the household, including the ability to care for children, the availability and consumption of food, and the overall quality of life. Finally, the study shows that there are communal sanctions on the use of remittances, especially when the receiver does not apply them toward household food needs. The food quest, cash remittances, and kin fosterage are major factors that contribute to an analysis of the social relations between village residents and their nonresident relatives.

THE RESEARCH AND SETTING

Data on which this paper is based were collected between September 1979 and May 1980 in Lisurnia, pseudonym for a Garifuna village in southern Belize (Palacio 1982). Methods of data collection included participant observation and informal and formal interviewing. Formal interviewing included a survey of food items consumed in almost all of the sixty-four households in the village. The data were collected on two different days using the twenty-four-hour recall method. The interviewing was carried out over three months (from January to April 1980); the days for which information was collected for each household were separated by some weeks.

Located in an area that has seen hardly any of the development efforts taking place in other parts of Belize during the past three decades, Lisurnia has the typical features of a marginal community. It is geographically isolated, being accessible only by a one-hour ride on powered dories from the nearest town along the Caribbean coast. It has a skeletal population of 250, consisting largely of children up to fourteen years old (63 percent) and older folk at least fifty years of age (24 percent). The remaining 13 percent are men and women aged fifteen to forty-nine, most of whom returned some years ago from doing wage labor in other parts of the country and abroad. The complete reliance on the outside world is reinforced by the self-fulfilling folk belief that children have to leave the village to acquire their livelihood.

KIN TIES AND FOSTERAGE

Kin ties are pervasive in Lisurnia, the village having been founded during the latter half of the nineteenth century by a few closely related men and women. Lisurnians distinguish between two sets of relatives, based on the recognition of closeness of blood ties and the subsequent obligations that are exercised. At one level there are *iduhenyu diseguaña* (distant relatives), who are persons originating remotely within one's patriline or matriline and with whom one does not readily enter into exchange relationships. For Lisurnians this category includes almost everyone in the village, since there are overlapping kin ties that they all share. At a more intimate level there are one's *iduhenyu carnal* (relatives of the flesh). They are one's immediate family members and close collaterals, the siblings of one's father and mother and their children. In contrast to the ambivalence in the relationship among *iduhenyu diseguaña*, that among *iduhenyu carnal* is well defined as the reference group for the exchange of material and other benefits.

The parent–child (father/mother–son/daughter) bond among the Garifuna is the highest level in the expression of kinship obligations among the *iduhenyu carnal*. A cardinal rule of conduct between parents and children is spelled out in the saying, "Thou shall *agriaha* thine children." The stem for *agriaha* comes from the verb meaning "to give birth to," "to nourish an infant," or "to sustain it with life-giving support." At the root of these synonyms is the need to feed someone as a part of providing him or her with the necessities of life, a process referred to as *agriahouni*. As a child grows to adulthood, the responsibilities of *agriahouni* become reversed, with the grown son or daughter having to contribute to the support of his or her parents.

In the Garifuna definition of the roles of parent and child there is a hierarchy of pivotal, relevant, and peripheral characteristics (Nadel 1956). The pivotal characteristic of *agriaha* is physically to give birth; a relevant characteristic is to feed someone as an aspect of giving them life-giving support. The care-giving aspect of the roles is generalized (namely, peripheral), can be shared by several persons, and is the basis of fosterage. The Garifuna term for fosterage is *agriahouni*, and the obligations of fosterage are expressed in terms of those between biological parents and children.

In the event that biological parents are unable to carry out their *agriahouni* obligations to their offspring, *iduhenyu carnal* (and sometimes other kin) can take over within the chain of reciprocal exchange (Sahlins 1965) that is ever present among them. This can occur for a brief period of some weeks or can extend to several years. It is done with the understanding that the child retains ties with the biological parents and that the care givers are acting only as surrogates. The biological ties between the senders of children and their keepers in Lisurnia are between women and close relatives in sixty-three cases (72 percent) and between men with close relatives in twenty-three cases (26 percent) (see Table 6.1). The fact that a little more than one-fourth of the cases are between men and their relatives is worth emphasizing, since there is usually little focus on Garifuna men in the literature on interactions among relatives.[1]

Until thirty or forty years ago parents left children for short periods while they were away seasonally at work sites or at swidden fields in surrounding communities; or sometimes they sent children to perform specific tasks for their close kin. Today fosterage is more widespread, and most boys and girls stay in the village with their caretakers for most of their childhood. Among the forty-three households with children in Lisurnia, thirty-two have children in fosterage, and the eighty-eight children in fosterage (Table 6.1) con-

T A B L E 6.1

Biological Relationship of the Senders of Children to the Keepers

Type	Number of Children
1. Mother's mother and father	30
2. Father's mother	14
3. Mother's mother	13
4. Father's father and mother	7
5. Mother's mother's sister	6
6. Mother's mother's mother	6
7. Mother's father's mother	3
8. Mother's sister	3
9. Distant relative of the mother	2
10. Father's mother's sister	1
11. Father's brother and father's sister-in-law	1
12. Mother's mother and mother's brother	1
13. Mother's father	1
Total	88

stitute about 60 percent of all children up to fourteen years and older in the village.

Fosterage is the means by which mothers and fathers who are working elsewhere arrange for the care of their children when they have to send them back to the village. The children, in turn, help in their keepers' households and play an indispensable role in all phases of subsistence production and food exchange. Boys and girls do chores in the gardens, planting and harvesting crops and carrying them home on their backs. They are needed to bring in firewood and buckets of water from the well. Boys catch fish for food on Saturdays and school holidays and may be paid for such errands as bringing luggage from the wharf for those arriving from town. Finally, children are the carriers of food items exchanged, and girls aged ten to thirteen may do their own petty trading of sweets at the schoolyard, preparing merchandise with help from other members of the household.

Remittances sent for the care of the children (usually as cash from outside Belize, and including food, clothing, and medicines from inside the country) also contribute to the welfare of other household members. These remittances often meet a dual obligation of *agriahouni*—toward both the children and the parents of the absent men and women.

THE SOCIOECONOMY OF FOOD

The food survey recorded the items consumed in the three daily meals eaten in Lisurnia and the source of the items. The classification used in the survey closely followed the folk system of subdividing foods (Palacio 1982, 1983), including the categories of beverage, bread, vegetable crop, meat, fish, seed crops, and dairy products.

Meals

Breakfast and supper are referred to respectively as a warm drink had in the morning (*bachati le lanina binafi*) and a warm drink

T A B L E 6.2
Frequently Recorded Food Items

Breakfast and Supper

Beverage
Coffee	boiled and left to steep
Milo	(malt-flavored powder)
	boiled and left to steep
Bush tea	(different leaves, barks, and roots)
	boiled and left to steep

Bread
| *Fein* | wheat-flour dough mixed with yeast and baked |
| *Durudia* | wheat-flour dough mixed with baking powder and roasted |

Fish
| *Furidu* | fried fish |

Dinner

Beverage
| Cool Aid | powder mixed in water and sweetened with sugar |

Vegetable crop
Rice	cooked with fat
Tapou	boiled green banana
Hudut	boiled green plantain, mashed

Fish
Falmou	fish boiled in coconut milk
Dunouti	fish boiled in water
Tikin	fish simmered in soup made by frying flour and adding water

had late in the afternoon (*bachati le lanina rambaweyu*), although no meal is considered complete without a combination of liquids and solids. Only dinner, the main meal, usually eaten at midday, is referred to by the word *eigini* (*eigini le lanina amidirugu*), a generic term for food that has been prepared and is ready to eat. And only at dinner are vegetable crops and more elaborate preparations of fish or other *uwi* eaten. Table 6.2 shows the most frequently recorded items for the different meals. Solids are divided into *uwi* (meat) and *breadkind* (filler—literally, something that fills up an empty space). The *uwi* is sometimes referred to as *leiganana* (the most essential part) of the dinner. The significance of *uwi* (which is usually fish) is underlined by the fact that its availability determines the timing of meal preparation. The chores of the housewife revolve around the arrival of the fishermen with their fresh catch; she waits to see if she can purchase some fish before hurrying home to cook the midday meal.

Differences between households in what they eat, and in the same household over time, reflect changes introduced by the housewife (to avoid monotony, or for Sundays and special occasions), seasonal fluctuations, and differential access to resources. For example, during the rainy season stormy weather makes fishing in small dories risky, and shopkeepers stock such items as canned meats and pickled pigtails, which the villagers buy. Fish, however, is generally available at least two or three times a week. But whereas Lisurnians readily accept fish as a main ingredient for all their meals, they are reluctant to eat rice daily. Older folk in particular complain that it is too light to provide the bulk the belly needs: They would prefer to have green bananas, plantains, and root crops more often. However, these are not as easily available as rice. Lisurnians are eating what they can get and not what they would like. This is especially ironic for a community that could produce most of the vegetable crops, among other foods, that it would want.

Sources of Food

Another objective of the food survey was to learn how household residents procure their food supply. There were three main possibilities—cash bought, home produced, and received through reciprocal exchange. Men, women, and children have different methods of acquiring cash and food (see Table 6.3).

Most foods are purchased at retail shops in the village and the town. The beverage ingredients in Table 6.2 and the bleached wheat flour used in the breads are imported into the country, and rice is shipped in from other parts of Belize. During periods of scarcity,

T A B L E 6.3
Methods of Food Acquisition

Sources of Cash	Use of Natural Resources	Reciprocal Exchange
Nonlocal sources	Land	Labor
Remittances M W C[a]	Clearing M	Fishing M
Salaries and pensions M	Cultivation W C	Cultivation W C
Public-work projects M		Food
Fish sales in town M		processing W C
Local sources	Sea	Role obligations
Odd jobs M	Fishing M	M W C
Lottery sales M W	Collecting	
Rum sales W	shelfish W C	
Fish sales M		
Food sales M W C		

[a]The initials M W C (men, women, children) signify who most often participates in a given activity.

corn and root crops are used as substitutes for wheat and plantains, and bananas or root crops take the place of rice; they are purchased at the town market or from traders in neighboring communities. To a very limited extent, root crops are also produced locally. Fish, the only item that is exclusively a village product, is also available to most villagers through purchase. It is sometimes replaced by other items, such as pork, bought from traveling traders.

More than thirty years ago there was greater local production of food through cultivation in swidden fields and fishing on banks off the coast. Changes in the local economy occurred when men and then women left in large numbers during the 1950s for wage labor in lumber camps, plantations, and factories in adjoining districts. Since the 1960s, they have gone further afield within the country and abroad, although they return for periods lasting from weeks to months for visits or when they are between jobs. Generally, men and women come back permanently when they are too old for the job market. Unfortunately, at such an age they do not have the strength to maintain swidden fields and to fish on a large scale, as had been done earlier.

Cash now enters the village economy primarily from sources in the rest of the country and overseas. It comes from remittances, and also from salaries and pensions, government subsidies for local public works projects, and the sale of fish in the town market. Men earn salaries and pensions, receive wages from public works projects, and sell fish. Women usually receive remittances, even when they do not head the household.

Apart from the all-important remittances, and the sale of fish, cash enters the village economy through three institutions. These are the village council, the credit union, and the church–school system, which also serve as linkages among Lisurnians and between them and the outside world. The main contribution of the village council to the economy is as an intermediary for subsidies from the central government to carry out village public works projects. The credit union is a savings and loan association that includes as members resident and nonresident Lisurnians. The church–school system educates children, preparing them for work opportunities in the outside world. Teaching is one such work opportunity. Among the forty men twenty years of age and older, eight are earning salaries and pensions. An additional three unmarried schoolteachers working in surrounding villages regularly send remittances to their parents. Five men sell fish once or twice weekly in the town market. On an average, the amount one of them earns during the month is less than that of one of the schoolteachers. Besides, their earnings are unpredictable, depending on fishing luck, the weather, and the demand for fish. The other twenty-four men do not have any steady income, but rely on various local opportunities for earning cash.

Locally, cash circulates through the sale of imported food items at two shops, the performance of such odd jobs as carpentry, and the petty sales of rum, lottery tickets, fish, household necessities (kerosene, matches), and homemade foods (bread, pastry, and sweets). Women, helped by children, do most of the petty trading. They engage in it merely as *murusu agarabahani* (turning over a little pittance)—something that can help with the basic household needs during intervals in the arrival of larger amounts from outside sources. Most villagers, men and women alike, maximize their interactions with absent persons, usually *iduhenyu carnal*, who can send them cash remittances, and it is on these remittances that the security of their food supply depends.

There is abundant land surrounding the village that is fit for cultivation. However, working it becomes a constant struggle against the perennial weeds and wild animals that destroy crops. It is estimated that for the whole village about five acres are being cultivated, mostly by about twenty women. They maintain plots adjoining each other to minimize the loss that each suffers from animal predators. The women complain that men are reluctant to clear the fields. They are forced to use the same plots and work even harder only to receive lesser yields from the depleted soil. Because of these problems, women turn their attention to tending crops in their house lots. Along with fruit trees (coconuts, citrus, golden plum, avocado, breadfruit, and the like) traditionally grown in lots, one increasingly sees such crops as cassava and other tubers that were previously confined to the swidden fields.

Potentially, there are greater returns available through fishing for home supply and for sale than from crop growing. But profitable fishing requires investment in gill nets, large dories, and outboard motors, which is only possible for someone with earnings from other previous employment. The man who catches the most fish uses such equipment. Four or five others who sell fish go out once or twice a week using the basic dory, paddle, and sail. Others fish occasionally for home use but not for sale.

The overwhelming obstacles that women encounter in their attempts to maintain fields and that men face in their attempts to fish limit their access to the two natural resources that are abundantly available. Lisurnians use other methods to supplement their food supply. One is to engage in indigenous forms of exchange relations. Working in pairs or groups in their fields and in the processing of food, women share in the product according to their contribution. Making cassava bread is a complex and labor-intensive undertaking that needs some collective effort and the use of implements that only a few women presently maintain; in return, the participants receive cassava bread. Men do likewise, borrowing dories and fishing gear in exchange for fish. Others take care of houses and lots for absent relatives in exchange for access to the fruit trees in the lots.

To participate in these forms of exchange it is necessary to be able to do the required work or to have implements that can be borrowed. Men and women who cannot work because of age or disability, or who lack implements because they have few material resources, rely on food exchange that is based solely on the role obligations of *iduhenyu carnal*. A son or a daughter sends cooked food to an aging mother, as does a sister to an ailing brother. Seven recipients (older men and women living by themselves) rely entirely on such food donations. These are persons whose food supply is most vulnerable, and who may finally have to rely on role obligations based on friendship and the status of *liliana fulasu* (fellow villager).

Other categories of people may also, though intermittently, rely on role obligations for supplementing their food supply in times of need; sisters and other close relatives frequently exchange small amounts of cooked food. But essentially, the main way of meeting daily food needs is by having cash. In other words, for the vast majority of Lisurnians having cash is not one source for food among several others: Without it one cannot eat.

Food and Rank

Control of access to food and observed food use are important bases and indicators of rank in Lisurnia, since neighbors can see what others bring home to cook. Those who are higher ranking have a relatively steady supply of food and can eat on time, not having to depend on daily fluctuations in the village supply. They vary staples to avoid monotony and maintain a mix of imported and home-produced foods. Additionally, these persons may boast of the attributes of their diet loudly so people can hear (Palacio 1982).

At the other end of the scale are those who suffer from food scarcity. They rely primarily on role obligations to get daily meals. In the absence of *iduhenyu carnal* they turn to other relatives or to those who are sympathetic to their plight. The villagers grumble about these persons, suggesting reasons why they have ended up this way—"They are suffering because they didn't have children or they didn't care for them properly." But the main reason for their criticism is that they feel some form of moral responsibility to help, since all villagers are related as *iduhenyu diseguaña*, although their own resources are already being strained. Their usual pattern of intervention is to make representation to negligent sons and daughters on meeting with them while traveling away from the village. In addition, the chairman of the village council or others with strong affiliations to the ruling political party may ask the Social Development Department officer to extend welfare assistance to some households.

MEN, WOMEN, AND CHILDREN IN THE HOUSEHOLD

The workings of households reveal the ongoing processes that link widespread kin ties; fosterage; the local socioeconomy; and the roles of men, women, and children in acquiring and using resources for the provision of necessities, including food. The word for house is *muna*, and the occupants are collectively referred to as *tilana muna* (those living in one house), a term denoting the group identity they share by virtue of residence.

Almost half of the households in Lisurnia are extended family households, where a relative(s) other than a child of either husband or wife is present. The remainder are divided equally between conjugal family (parent[s] and children) and single-person households; one other household is occupied by a brother and sister (see Table 6.4). Twelve of the sixteen conjugal family households contain younger men and women with four or more of their children. Three are spouses without children, and one is a widowed mother with children. For the purposes of this study the extended family households were divided into two basic categories, based on the predominance of collateral or descent ties among the occupants. Extended family households may, usually for relatively

T A B L E 6.4
Household Types
(Based on Consanguineal and Affinal Ties Among Occupants)

	Number	Percentage of Total
Sibling	1	1.50
Single-person	16	25.00
Conjugal family	16	25.00
Extended family—collateral	4	6.25
Extended family—descent		
three-generation	22	34.40
four-generation	4	6.25
five-generation	1	1.60
Total	64	100.0

short periods, become multiple family households with more than one resident conjugal family (see, for example, the case discussion of the Juana Lopez household later in this chapter).

Four extended family households are characterized by collateral kinship. In three cases, the residents include a woman as head living with children whose mother is her sister or a close relative. In one the head is a fifty-one-year-old woman who is caring for two of her younger sister's children, twelve and six years of age. She is childless, while her sister is burdened with eight children in poor, overcrowded conditions in Belize City. Both the resident children, especially the twelve-year-old, are helpful to their aunt. Besides being messengers for the selling of homemade bread and sweets, they produce root crops in their house lot. The other three women with the same type of extended families find themselves in similar conditions. They do not have any younger children of their own and have taken as substitutes the children of relatives, thereby relieving them of some of their own child-rearing problems.

The kind of fosterage in these households is atypical, both in the biological relationships between the care giver and the children and in the underlying social relations. They do depict, however, two common features of fosterage that are found in all cases. One is that it is a part of the exchange of favors among *iduhenyu carnal*. The other is that fosterage allows access to the services of children that are so essential for the working and survival of the household.

The vast majority of extended family households span three generations (see Table 6.4). In four households descent extends to the fourth generation, and in one to the fifth. Among residents of the second, third, and subsequent generations there are varying degrees of collateral ties, including siblings, cousins, and aunts and uncles/nieces and nephews. In terms of food supply and overall well-being, the significance of fosterage in households featuring descent kinship spanning two or more generations is that it increases the possibility of the care giver's receiving remittances that contribute to meeting both the needs of the children and their own needs.

There are only thirty out of the sixty-four households in which both spouses are present; in all the others the men and women are either widowed or permanently separated. Men do not migrate and leave their wives to care for their children in the village. The relationship between spouses can best be described using the Garifuna distinctions. The man is referred to as *tabuti muna* (the leader or head of the household), the woman as *tabureme muna* (owner or manager of the household). These terms depict two areas of responsibility essential for the upkeep of the village household. Other household members, once they are old enough, are helpers within the household, particularly helpers of women.

Men are seen as the main source of authority, particularly in making major decisions involving outsiders. Extreme examples of this arise during moments of crisis in illness and death. Because of this position, they are shown particular respect and served first at meals. In economic matters their most important contribution is cash. They also have household-related chores to perform, which include chopping the grass and repairing the house and furniture, as well as clearing the garden and fishing; when the women are unable to do so, they may also prepare the food.

As the people primarily responsible for managing the household and as the ones concerned with its daily operation, women have diverse tasks to perform, including cooking, cleaning, and child care, as well as the food- and cash-acquiring activities described earlier. They also have to try to fill in when men and children do not carry out their duties adequately. It is they who are finally expected to see that there is food for the household, and they serve themselves only when they have served everyone else. An efficient housewife is one who consistently maintains an adequate food supply, namely, enough to feed her household three times a day. In doing this women make use of a wider range of food acquisition opportunities in the village than do men. They engage extensively in reciprocal exchange, and they link their cultivation and household chores with petty trading, selling foodstuffs that they produce. In all these activities, they are helped by older children. Although ideally the responsibilities of men and women in the household are complementary, the wide range of activities of women in both the domestic and extradomestic realms makes it easier for them to head households without spouses. But without spouses, remittances and the help of children are even more important.

The differential use of cash by men and women highlights their household responsibilities. Women buy more items than do men; men spend on rum, cigarettes, and fishing gear; and both spend on food, lottery tickets, and sweets (see Table 6.5). With respect to food, men limit their purchases to such staples as flour, sugar, and rice and do so irregularly. They may buy a week's supply on Saturday with proceeds from fish sales in the town. Women either maintain direct responsibility for food buying or send children to purchase the supplies they need. When men do not go to town to sell fish they do not buy the weekly groceries. Women buy food items almost daily from the village shops. Next to food, savings are the major source of cash expenditure for women. They have four main outlets—the credit union, a rotating credit association, a women's group affiliated with one of the national political parties, and saving at home (Palacio 1982).

Women's role in saving reflects both their often limited access to cash and their need to supply the household with food, irrespective of fluctuations in food supplies in the village and in their own households. Since women save secretly, in their homes or under

T A B L E 6.5
Items on Which Men and Women Spend Cash, Based on Data for
One Month

	Men	Women
Food	X	X
Household goods		
Clothes		X
School supplies		X
Toiletry		X
Kerosene		X
Savings		X
Recreation		
Rum	X	
Lottery	X	X
Sweets	X	X
Cigarettes	X	
Hardware goods		
Machete	X	
Fishing gear	X	

their own names in various sorts of savings funds (there are no joint savings accounts for women and men), they can have considerable independence in controlling their use of cash. A woman can always claim that she does not have any more money to buy food; her spouse, ignorant of the amount she actually has, may believe her. It becomes a strategy that she can use to demand money, not only to use in the short run, but also to keep for a "rainy day." A high value is placed on frugality, and women strive to spend as little money as they can on food, obtaining as much as possible from other sources. The emphasis on frugality is also seen in relation to food consumption: One should avoid extravagance in eating, and there is a nickname for those who are known as big eaters.[2]

Whether or not women succeed through their many and varied activities in providing their households regularly with sufficient food of the sort they wish to have will depend to a great extent on the degree to which others are able to, and do, fulfill their obligations to provide them with cash and food. It will also depend on the composition of the household. The members of young conjugal households who cannot expect to receive remittances and who have no steady source of cash appear particularly vulnerable, especially when they also have a number of small children and no older children to help them with their many domestic and income-generating activities. The consequences are particularly evident for those children who should be receiving supplementary food and for those who are being weaned. In Lisurnia economic limitations in terms of the household food supply have a greater effect on the feeding of small children than beliefs about what is or is not suitable for eating (Palacio 1982).

Potentially, extended households should be in a better position, with older children to help, few children at the critical weaning stage, and remittances for the care of the members of the household and the children they are fostering. But in practice those who should send remittances fulfill the obligations of *agriahouni* toward their two sets of dependents—their children and their parents—only to varying degrees. This can be seen from the social and economic conditions within the household and through the reactions of the village community. The case studies that follow provide examples.

Juana Lopez Household

Juana lives with her ten grandchildren and three great-grandchildren (see Figure 6.1). Six of the grandchildren are those of her son, who lives in Chicago, and the other four are her daughter's, who died two years ago. Her oldest granddaughter is temporarily in the village to give birth to her third child.

Juana no longer keeps a bush plot of her own. Her income consists of regular cash remittances from her son and an allowance of about Bze $100.[3] per month from the government on behalf of her deceased daughter. She attends to sick women and children with bush medicine, for which she receives donations of food and cash. Occasionally, she processes cassava bread with her friends and relatives, receiving some in return. Her oldest granddaughter

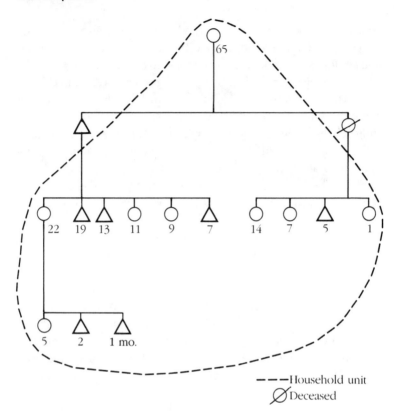

F I G U R E 6.1
The Juana Lopez Household

brought cash to contribute toward her keep, as well as that of her children. Almost all the daily chores, including caring for the younger children, are done by the older boys and girls. Juana's role is that of supervising them and of managing the household resources.

Juana is responsible for ascertaining the flow of income from different sources and the allocation. She periodically checks with the Social Development Department in the town about the allowance for her late daughter's children and keeps up communication with her son and granddaughter. In this regard, she receives help from the older boys and girls, who can more easily make trips to the town to call their father in Chicago by telephone.

The children in Juana's household appear as well and healthy as most of the village children, despite the fact that they make up the largest number in any one household. Generally, the villagers attribute this to Juana's good fortune in having offspring who care for her and for their children.

Martha Castillo Household

This household presents a contrast to that of Juana, particularly in not receiving remittances. Martha is living with four grandchildren from two sons, and two great grandchildren (Figure 6.2). The main source of livelihood comes from a small salary that her grand-

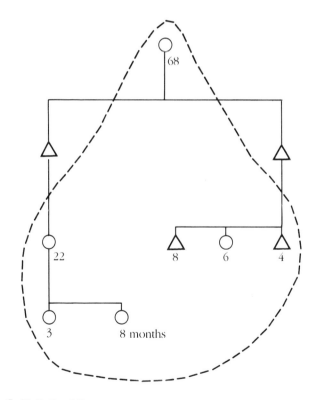

F I G U R E 6.2
The Martha Castillo Household

daughter Lorna earns as a lower-grade teacher in the village school; she expects to remain in Lisurnia for a few more months. Lorna's salary, which is barely sufficient to meet her living expenses together with that of her own children, contributes minimally to the keep of the other household members. The father of the other three grandchildren (ages eight, six, and four) has not sent anything to his mother for several months. He lives in a town in northern Belize with his own family.

Martha has been sickly for the past few years; as a result, she has not been able to maintain a bush plot or to do petty trading. She often goes to a niece's house to ask for food, pills, kerosene, and other necessities. The niece obliges, but not always with a willing heart. Martha grumbles that the niece is the only one on whom she can rely and that she should help her, since Martha had cared for her as a child.

The children, especially the three young grandchildren, are also sick most of the time with colds, sores, and diarrhea. In appearance they are the most unhealthy and malnourished in the village. A few months before I arrived one of them had died from an illness diagnosed as kwashiorkor in the town hospital.[4] The extremely deprived conditions in Martha Castillo's household have taken their toll in the death of her grandchild. The villagers deliver their verdict on the cause of Martha's misfortune: On becoming incapacitated she was neglected by her two sons, although she is caring for the children of one.

Martha herself admitted to me that she knew that with her physical disabilities she would not be able to care for younger children. But she hoped that having the children would increase her chances of receiving support from their father, who had neglected her for years. There are few women with Martha's disadvantages who are caring for children; generally, the care givers are more capable than she is. In many fosterage cases both men and women are looking after children (see Table 6.1). There is a selectivity being exercised by the parents of children who prefer not to send them to such women as Martha. Unfortunately, this also decreases their chances of receiving remittances, worsening their miserable condition. As a last resort, they may leave the village to join their children or move in with sympathetic relatives.

Peter Martinez Household

The Martinez household contrasts with that of Martha Castillo in having access to remittances, but the overall conditions are hardly better.

Peter and his wife live with four of their grandchildren from their two sons and one daughter (see Figure 6.3), who are all in New York. Their main source of livelihood is a monthly remittance of $300 Bze. received on behalf of one of the grandsons from their daughter. The money comes from the U.S. federal government on

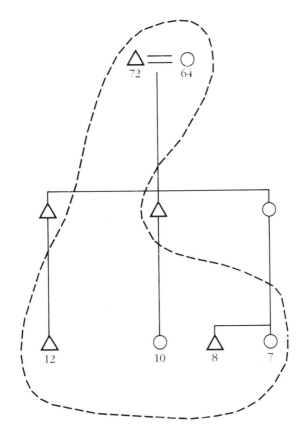

F I G U R E   6.3
The Peter Martinez Household

behalf of the child's father, a veteran of the armed forces. The two sons send cash regularly. Peter and his wife also engage in fishing and cultivation.

However, unlike his wife, Peter is not conscientious in carrying out his household responsibilities—on collecting the cash at the town post office, he goes on binges for days on end. From the small amount he gives to his wife, he demands money to buy rum later in the month. His wife left the village for a time while I was there; Peter's drinking problem worsened and, along with it, the care that the children received.

The villagers unanimously disapprove of Peter's behavior. Comments I heard about him included "He should spend that money to buy food for his grandchildren," and "He should bear in mind the hard work that his children perform to earn that money, which he is spending so foolishly." One villager even sent letters to one of his sons to inform him about Peter's unfatherly behavior. Although the son came and admonished his father, Peter shortly resumed his heavy drinking.

In analyzing the linkage between remittances and fosterage from the viewpoint of Lisurnians, there is conceptually a "correct fit," as seen in the overall quality of life in the household. Some indices include the food consumed and the health and welfare of the children, the ability to meet daily living responsibilities, and the level of harmony among household members (and between them and relatives who are away). But there are constraints on the working of the ideal situation.

One concerns the level of *hatuadi* (physical activity) of the carer. For women it connotes being able to perform one's household chores, including various food acquisition and child care tasks. The worst possibility is to leave children with a person who is ailing, as in the case of Martha. Another constraint is the age range of the children. It is difficult for older women to care for younger children, who themselves cannot contribute to the welfare of the household. The situation improves when there are children old enough to take over the care of younger ones. One of the differences between the Juana Lopez and Martha Castillo households is that in the former there are several older children who can assume responsibilities for household chores. Of course, it is essential that the biological parents send remittances. The consensus is that remittances should come at regular intervals as well as in response to crisis situations.

Finally, the burden is on the person receiving the remittances to use them for the daily needs of the household members. When this is not done, the villagers criticize the care giver for reneging on his or her responsibilities toward the children as well as toward their biological parents. Such foster parents are not living up to their *agriahouni* obligations—to help their children and to care for their children's children.

SUMMARY AND CONCLUSION

In arguing that behavior related to food can lead to an analysis of the maintenance of kin ties, and thus to an understanding of how the norms and relationships of kinship define how food is acquired and used, I have combined the use of concepts that are usually treated separately. These are the socioeconomy of food, fosterage, and remittances.

The discussion on the socioeconomy of food is necessary to illustrate the relative importance of the different kinds of food acquisition methods in Lisurnia. Having multiple ways to obtain food is important in a rural community that uses a wide variety of methods, some of which do not fall into the traditional dichotomy of subsistence and cash economies. Although most of the food eaten is purchased, not all of it comes from the cash-earning activities of the villagers. A strict costing of food items would tell us what is bought, for how much, and what is not bought. We do need to know, however, how items that are bought and not bought enter the household. We can thus appreciate the importance of reciprocal exchange of food through the use of materials and services and through role obligations between relatives. It sets the stage for subsequent discussion of the receipt of remittances by those caring for children, which essentially is a form of reciprocal exchange for food (or cash with which to buy food) based on role obligations.

A discussion of the socioeconomy of food also leads to an insight into the village social organization. The use of food is a marker of one's status in the village system of social stratification. Food behavior indicates the importance of cash, the social pressures that exist to get it, and the ways in which those who are without it are regarded.

The concept of kin fosterage among Lisurnians revolves around the transfer of rights and obligations from biological parent and child to foster parent and child, while those between the biological parent and child remain (Goody 1978). It includes the maintenance of a series of dyadic ties that fit into the life cycle of those participating, resulting in a person being able to rely on another for the provision of basic needs, especially food (referring to the use of the Garifuna concept of *agriahouni*). Kin fosterage, therefore, has a long-term dimension analogous to that of working as a paid employee with the expectation of receiving a retirement pension to help during one's old age.

In discussing remittances I am concerned with their connections to fosterage. In extended family households where fosterage is based on collateral kinship, there is little expectation of remittances. There is expectation of it in extended family households that include as foster children one's lineal descendants. The coupling of remittances with fosterage, resulting in meeting household needs, is an ideal that is not always realized. Those who are supposed to send funds may not; the children need to be within the age range during which the provision of care is not excessively demanding; and the carer has to be physically capable of meeting the challenge of village life, including being able to acquire what the household needs other than exclusively through remittances. Finally, the community places sanctions on what it considers to be the appropriate use of remittances.

Most of the literature on remittances stresses the use of cash for the benefit of the sender in preparing for retirement (Watson 1977) or the welfare of the recipients in acquiring material possessions that they could not otherwise afford (Lord 1975). Chaney's (1985) exhaustive review of the literature on remittances, among other aspects of Caribbean migration, concludes that household consumption needs and house construction are the two most common uses of remittances. Investment of cash remittance in capital goods and related commodities in Lisurnia is minimal. Its most significant use is to care for the daily needs of care givers and children.

Ultimately, food behavior in Lisurnia confirms the strength of the parent/child bond among kinfolk and between fathers and children as well as between mothers and children. The emphasis on carrying through with the culturally defined obligations rests on the economic conditions in which Lisurnians find themselves. Since they cannot provide for their daily livelihood in the village, they emigrate to job sites where they find conditions that prevent them from bringing along their children. As a result, they leave them with relatives. Furthermore, there are men and women who for various other reasons do not care for their own offspring. In such cases, a relative may take over as a foster parent and establish a dyadic relationship with all the rights and obligations that accompany those of biological parenthood.

The future of fosterage in Lisurnia depends, on the one hand, on the problems that deter the villagers from settling with their families at the work sites and, on the other, on whether there are men and women in the home village who can take care of children. Already there are cases where men and women are too old to offer such care. If they are not replaced by new returnees, there will be no one to nurture children. This will end a practice that is entrenched in Lisurnia and will also hasten the demise of the village as a community.

NOTES

Acknowledgments: The research was funded by the Inter-American Foundation under its Doctoral Program for the Study of Social Change.

1. The focus on parent and child relationships in the Caribbean literature is dominated by the concepts of legitimacy and matrifocality. Whitehead (1978) is unusual in studying the roles of men as fathers in a Jamaican

town by looking at the incidence of food donations between them and the mothers of their children.

2. The emphasis on frugality in consumption within the household is in marked contrast to the large amounts of food considered appropriate for village festivities (Palacio 1982).

3. The exchange rate for the Belize dollar was Bze. $1.00 = U.S. $0.50 in 1979 and 1980.

4. Martha attributed the sickness and death to food use—not to the lack of food, but to *umou* (the belief that some species of large fish emanate certain odors that can harm those with a weak constitution, such as infants).

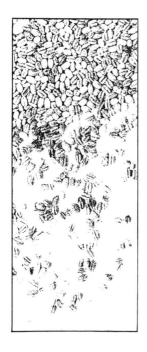

CHAPTER 7

Sisters, Mothers, and Daughters: Food Exchange and Reciprocity in an Italian-American Community

Janet Theophano

Karen Curtis

The research on which Janet Theophano and Karen Curtis's contribution is based was designed in part to study the relation between ethnicity and dietary practices through the study of Italian Americans. In this it represents a development in the analysis of food as an aspect of culture in the tradition of Mead (1943) and other cultural anthropologists. But in defining their subject of study and in collecting and analyzing their data, they have also drawn on other traditions in anthropology. They have created their own approach, established new ways of looking at food and diet, and raised issues concerning diet and domestic life in society that need to be explored further, particularly the question of the importance of social network analysis.

For studying dietary practices (and innovation, variation, and conservatism in diets), they have shown the importance of looking at both daily and festive events and interactions and at the whole chain of food related activities from procurement through cooking, eating, and disposal. They have also developed a way of analyzing different levels in a food system and have placed food exchange and reciprocity in the context of exchange of other goods and services.

Although households are important units of study in their work, Theophano and Curtis recognized early on that the community which they studied could be seen as a series of women's articulated personal networks, defined to a considerable extent by food exchange and reciprocity. They selected households with different characteristics and from different parts of the community by tracing out these networks. Their contribution to this book focuses on one social network composed of women of several generations in varying relationships to one another. Theophano and Curtis analyze households and social networks as being continually created and redefined through different kinds of food exchange and reciprocity, and they show the history of these units and the experiences of their members as generating particular family traditions and patterns of food consumption.

In anthropology there is a long tradition of studying food exchange, reciprocity, and distribution. These processes symbolize and constitute social relationships. They may be used to maintain social position and to extend spheres of influence. Food exchange, which varies from household to household even within a given culture, can contribute to the provisioning of domestic and larger social units (Raymond Firth [1946] 1966; Sahlins 1965; Richards 1939). Research has largely been carried out, however, in relatively small-scale, sometimes quite isolated, nonindustrial societies; has often focused on the activities of men; and has not, in most cases, looked in detail at how these activities affect the diets of particular households. This chapter, by contrast looks at food exchange and reciprocity in a middle-class Italian-American community in a suburb of a large city. It focuses particularly on the way in which food exchange and reciprocity illuminate the continual redefinition of the household unit, domestic activities, and social relationships. It also looks at their consequences for innovation, variation and conservatism in diet, and for the provisioning of households.

Food exchange and its concomitant, reciprocity, is an integral aspect of the social life and the domestic organization of Italian Americans in the suburban community of Maryton (a pseudonym). Food is used as gifts, as contributions to shared family meals, and as payment for services, anticipated or completed. In this way, food acts as a link among families, networks, individuals, and generations. Food exchange and reciprocity are particularly the domain of women, and so also are activities through which women establish, maintain, and express their social positions. In this chapter food exchange and reciprocity are examined in a social network composed of several generations of women in varying relationships to one another. Of particular importance is food exchange between sisters, mothers, and daughters, which is examined here in relation to the domestic organization of the families of two women. These women were chosen as case studies because they are close in age, are the heads of single-parent households, and share similar contemporary life situations (including a close friendship), but at the same time have very different patterns of food exchange and reciprocity.

Analysis of a food system requires attention to both daily and festive events and interactions. It is through comparison and contrast with ritual occasions that everyday patterns reveal systematic behavior and interaction, including reciprocity. Ritual and festive food events symbolize and express the relationships of everyday life (Geertz 1973; Ortner 1978) and thus also constantly redefine and strengthen relationships that are important in more mundane circumstances and for more practical reasons. In this community, ritual serves (among its many functions) to make explicit the differentiation of sex roles and the shifting relationships among members of the network. Women are the guardians of domestic ritual, and decision making is largely in their hands. It is through the female network that decisions about ritual occasions are negotiated.

In this chapter, to show the relationship between ritual and everyday occasions, the periods selected for analysis are the week prior to Easter Sunday in the household of one woman and an ordinary week in the household of the other. These time frames also make it possible to trace the distribution of food items from their raw state to their ultimate designation as leftovers. Throughout both weeks, daily meals are occasions for daughters and sisters to visit and share a meal. After any extended family meal, leftovers are distributed according to the relationship to the hosting cook and the size of the family. Patterns described for the households of the two women in this chapter are similar to those of other households in the community, both with and without resident husbands or fathers.

RESEARCH METHODS AND PROCEDURES: DATA COLLECTION

The data for this chapter were obtained during two periods of fieldwork, in which varied techniques of data collection were used. The research effort profited from the multiple perspectives offered by the different kinds of data collected.

The first phase of the research focused on a section of Philadelphia. The data presented are from the second phase of the study, which involved intensive participant observation in the suburban community of Maryton.

The research was to involve observing and sharing the meals of four households, focusing on the observation of a household's kitchen, every day consecutively for one month, without interruption. For practical reasons we devised a schedule for the fieldwork in which the time spent in the community was shared; we tried to alternate days as much as possible. Having two fieldworkers enabled us to maintain the necessary continuity, since in case of illness or other personal crises coverage could be assured by one of the fieldworkers. We kept an account of every food variety and how it was prepared and served; and approximations were made about the amounts eaten by each individual. We were concerned with decor, table settings, seating arrangements, conversation at the table, cleanup, and length of time spent at the table. However, we were free to select other areas for observation. During ritual or festive events at which large numbers of guests were present, both of us could observe. This minimized lost time in the field and maximized coverage at any one time.

The situation of team fieldwork led to insights into another of the community's values—the attempt to be impartial and fair in the treatment of others. Everyone went to great lengths to make certain that both the researchers had the opportunity to taste the same foods, make the same breads and cookies, run the same errands, hear the same stories, and be invited to the same special occasions. Every effort was made to treat us impartially and as equals. The reality was that we ate different foods and were responded to as different and unique personalities. But the overall concern was to prevent disharmony and inequality of treatment. The differences in treatment of each fieldworker were based upon other criteria. One of us was married with a child (Theophano); the other was single (Curtis). These criteria cut beyond the level of ethnographer. The differences that were acknowledged did not have to do with personality, although these were recognized: It was the difference in life-style that was dealt with behaviorally. And this was the difference that helped us to learn something of the priority given to family life and social relationships as these were expressed in and through the food system.[1]

THE COMMUNITY

Maryton is a small industrial borough in the Philadelphia metropolitan area. Many of the residents are Italian Americans whose parents and grandparents immigrated from the same area in southern Italy. For two generations the women in this community have interacted with one another, initially due in part to residential segregation and the mutual aid efforts of immigrants dealing with unfamiliar situations. This early community developed its own business institutions and social and marital ties between residents that would continue to shape the lives of their descendants. Most recently, despite dispersed residential patterns and varying social mobility, the women voluntarily continue to maintain close family and friendship networks.

One of the ways in which the influence of the early community is felt is through the development of a food system that is shared, albeit transformed. The system is shared by the local network, which originated in the initial period of segregation.

SHARED COMMUNITY PATTERN

The food system is based on a dual classification of meal types, Italian (referred to as gravy and one-pots) and American (platters). The contemporary system, although expanded and more complex, is based on an immigrant pattern of alternation of one-dish meals with the segregated presentation of meat, fish, or eggs. The dual classification is the basis of a series of meal types and event formats that are constructed from elements of the weekly meal cycle arranged in new relationship. (See Tables 7.1 and 7.2 for weekly and festive-food formats.) This commensal cycle, rather than particular foods or spices, is the locus of continuity and intergenerational

T A B L E 7.1
Contemporary Weekly Meal Cycle

Meal	Weekday	Friday	Weekend	
Breakfast	Breakfast or partial breakfast	Breakfast or partial breakfast	Elaborate breakfast	
Lunch	Full lunch or abbreviated lunch	Full lunch or abbreviated lunch	Late and abbreviated lunch	
			Saturday	**Sunday**
Dinner	Gravy or platter	Fish or meatless, gravy or platter	"Noncooking" meal in home or celebratory eating out	Gravy and/or whole meat
Postdinner	Club, simple party, dessert and coffee	Late-night breakfast	Late-night breakfast	Dessert and coffee

transmission. Within the context of this shared community pattern, food exchange is demonstrative of and embedded in a set of domestic and social obligations and expectations among the members of the network.

Network Relationships

The members of this community are related to each other on several levels: social, economic, religious, and political. One or another level may become primary in different situations. Commitment to family, friends, and neighbors binds the community together. In the immigrant generation, residential proximity made it

T A B L E 7.2
Festive-Food Formats

Food-Event Type	Content	Service/ Consumption	Location	Attendance
Elaborated Sunday dinner	Gravy and whole meat	Two-plus courses; service and consumption at same table	In home	Extended family (10–15)
Buffet	Gravy and platter elements	Simultaneous presentation; self-service, consumption at several different tables	In or outside home	Extended family plus intimate and extended network (may be gender based) (50–125)
Buffet-style	Gravy and platter	Simultaneous presentation; self-service, consumption at one table	In home	Extended family (15–30)
Simple party	Appetizers, drinks, desserts	Simultaneous presentation; self-service, informal seating for consumption	In home	Extended family plus intimate network (may be gender based) (15–40)

T A B L E   7.2 (*continued*)

Food-Event Type	Content	Service/ Consumption	Location	Attendance
Sit-down catered dinner	Gravy of platter elements	Three-plus courses; service, consumption at same table	Outside home	Extended family plus intimate, extended, and work network (150-plus)

easy for women to exchange social information, child care, goods and services, gossip, and other mutual aid. Similarly, men were able to share and trade the products of their labors. As the children of immigrants emerged with new skills in carpentry, masonry, contracting, and plumbing, and with new roles as the full-time retail providers of goods, they were able to supply necessary skills and goods within a framework of trust and often reduced rates and charges that were reciprocated with favors, business referrals, and other gifts. Marriage and the birth of children reinforced the ties between family groups. Women continued to support domestic and social life through a network of mutual aid and exchange. In everyday life the bonds are demonstrated through the exchange of food.

Gender Roles and Women's Work

Social life in Maryton is predicated on gender differences. Women live under a set of life expectations and experience a body of knowledge that is centered on the family. Their roles are defined by responsibilities for shopping, cooking, child rearing, housekeeping, and nurturance of a wider family group and social network. These obligations are pervasive and primary, while professional aspirations are limited. When women work outside the home, which they often do, their work does not take them far or long from the house. Both of the women who are the focus of this study are employed. Anne's work takes her to a nearby community, where she cleans several families' houses, sharing these jobs with an older sister. Marcella is in charge of the county's local information office; it is within walking distance, and she manages to come home for lunch nearly every day. The majority (82 percent) of the women we worked with have full- or part-time jobs in the shops, offices, and light industries of the community. Employment is part of the system of sociability; proximity makes daily visiting and shared lunches possible, while the services and food involved in various occupations are shared among the group. Women in this community do not work at "careers," but at jobs. Their earnings supplement a husband's income (or other assistance in case of separation or divorce). Working outside the home takes place in the years before child bearing and after the children are grown. Women's primary work is to establish and maintain the families and friendship ties that secure them to the community.[2] Marriage and maternity are the essential markers of womanhood and the achievement of "full social recognition" (Perry 1978). The birth of the first child signals full adult status for both husband and wife. A woman who remains unmarried is denied the nurturing role of wife and mother, while an unmarried man may act as provider for an extended family, as would his married counterpart. Thus, the nurturing associated with maternity provides the model for analogous behavior as women interact in all of their social roles.

Generational Cohorts

The women we have worked with are members of a core generational cohort in the community. As the children of immigrants, they share common life experiences, involving the transition from poverty and segregation in their youth to an increased standard of living (and mobility) as adolescents and adults. They are in mid life; having raised their families, they now prepare for and enjoy the responsibilities of being grandparents.

Women in the mid-life cohort formed friendships in childhood and have maintained these ties throughout life. This group meets informally as members of such named associations as "Girls Club" and "Mah-Jongg Club." Few newcomers have been recruited into the circle since its members married in the early 1950s. The ties of friendship were augmented by marriages, which produced many affinal kinship relations as well. Following marriage and childbirth, women become more closely affiliated with their consanguineal and affinal female kin and age cohorts. This is not true for men, whose primary role is to provide for their conjugal family, while continuing to show concern for their natal families. A new family grouping is referred to by the name of the wife or mother, the maintainer of family ties. Although a wife's primary responsibilities are in her conjugal home, more time and energy are devoted to her female kin and network than before her marriage. The bond of female affiliation becomes more significant and is expressed through the intensified exchange of goods and services between families. Houses as well as families are identified with women, and attainment of their "own kitchens" imposes expectations for hospitality to an expanding network of family and friends.

TWO CASE STUDIES: MARCELLA AND ANNE

Two of the women of the mid-life cohort, Marcella Fiore and Anne Cooper, are the focus of this chapter. Marcella and Anne, friends for many years, act as extended family. Marcella's youngest daughter and Anne's son plan to marry after a courtship that began in high school.

Despite such family ties, each woman is in a different position in the social networks of Maryton. Marcella is a central figure in several social networks; her pivotal position is derived from several factors. First, she was born into a relatively prosperous and well-established family in Maryton. Second, she was reared and educated in the community. Marriage to a local Calabrese descendent strengthened her extended family ties. As an information broker employed by the county, Marcella meets new people and affirms old ties daily. Above all, she is an ebullient and gregarious personality and a doyenne of traditional cookery. This, no doubt, enables her to enlarge an already wide and solid network of family and friends.

Anne, in contrast, was raised in an impoverished working-class family and neighborhood. After her marriage to a local non-Italian, she achieved the material comforts and financial security she sought. Anne's social life revolves around her family—children and siblings (all sisters)—and several friends. She is not as active in as many social networks as Marcella, nor does she specialize in cooking. Rather, Anne takes great pride and excels in her ability to clean a house. Although she cooks plentifully for her family, this activity does not provide the same satisfaction and fascination she derives from tidying, washing, and dusting her home. She considers herself a homebody and prefers to interact with her family and close friends. This may, in part, account for her smaller network.

In addition to their divergent interests, the cooking repertoire of each woman is different. Marcella's specialty is "traditional" cookery: Kidney stew, *taralles*, homemade pasta, *pittacina, calamari*, and spaghetti are dishes for which she is noted. Friends and family depend on her to provide these foods for appropriate occasions, such as weddings, Christmas, and other celebratory events. Anne's preferences are for American "platters," soups, and stews. Neither her health nor her family's tastes would permit her to venture deeply into traditional Italian cooking.

Although both women are embedded in the Maryton Italian community, their standing in different networks and their unique personal and familial histories have contributed to differentiated household eating characteristics despite their shared community pattern.

Patterns of Exchange: The Fiores

To give some sense of the varieties and frequency of food exchange in this community, we shall recapitulate the events of the week preceding Easter, one that involved a flurry of eating and cooking activity. (See Figure 7.1 for a diagram of relationships among participants.)

Easter week begins with Palm Sunday. Supper on this evening

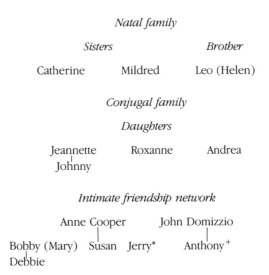

Marcella

Natal family

Sisters   *Brother*

Catherine   Mildred   Leo (Helen)

Conjugal family

Daughters

Jeannette   Roxanne   Andrea
|
Johnny

Intimate friendship network

Anne Cooper   John Domizzio
| |
Bobby (Mary) Susan Jerry*   Anthony⁺
|
Debbie

*Intended marriage to Andrea Fiore
⁺Intended marriage to Roxanne Fiore

F I G U R E 7.1
Major Participants in Exchange Activities: Relationship to Marcella

was a buffet-style dinner for about thirty people. The menu consisted of hot roast beef sandwiches, macaroni and ricotta, baked beans, salad, ambrosia, and strawberry shortcake. One of Marcella's sisters shared the cost of the roast beef, although Marcella prepared it. The same sister prepared and brought baked beans and the ambrosia for dessert. Another sister prepared her specialty (as she does for almost all occasions), macaroni and ricotta cheese.

Tuesday evening, Marcella's oldest daughter's fiancé was invited to dinner. He requested a special meatloaf filled with green beans and cheese.

Preparations for the special holiday foods began on Wednesday. In a cooperative effort, Marcella and her two sisters contributed the ingredients or shared the costs. An estimate was proposed of $5.50 per person for Easter breads (*pittalatte*); each person would receive three or four loaves. Marcella's sister Catherine brought ten pounds of flour, five pounds of sugar, nine dozen eggs, and a tuna hoagie to her sister's house. (The latter was to provide the energy Marcella would need for the baking.) In advance of the holiday, three Easter pies (called *pittacina*, and usually served after Good Friday) were made at the request of Marcella's daughter, who was eager to taste them. While the breads were baking, a few female relatives dropped in for wine, tea, and cake: Evenings of food preparation are usually occasions for socializing as well.

On Thursday, Marcella and Roxanne were invited to dinner at Catherine's house.

The primary occasion for preparing the pies was on Good Friday evening. The cost of the ingredients—pounds of assorted meats and cheeses, including Italian varieties—was calculated and shared among the three sisters (at $7.00 a person). About a dozen pies were prepared that evening to be shared among the family and given as gifts. In addition, Marcella's daughter made a special, less spicy meat pie for Anne's son, her fiancé.

Given her many culinary accomplishments, it is Marcella's sole responsibility to prepare the dough for the pies, as she did for the breads. While preparations were under way for the holiday baking (all of the women shared the labor of cutting the meats and cheeses into appropriate sizes), Marcella was also making a meatless Good Friday dinner for nine people.

The meatless dinner consisted of an asparagus *frittata* (a traditional Good Friday dish), monk fish, harvard beets, bread and butter (the bread was brought by Anne's son from an Italian bakery), wine, *pisadi* (a ricotta pizza), and a variety of desserts. Before the meal was eaten, a portion of it in the form of a platter was sent to one of Marcella's friends, who was working.

During the evening, other guests arrived to watch the baking activity and to visit. At midnight, following dinner, and with great anticipation, the meat pies were cut and served. Andrea's fiancé, who had brought the bread for dinner, took home his special pie and also an Easter bread for his mother, Anne Cooper.

Saturday morning, Marcella, Anne, and one of the researchers went out for breakfast at a nearby restaurant. Anne brought some rice pudding (one of her specialties) and *taralles* to Marcella. That afternoon, Marcella and her sister visited their brother for tea and cake.

Saturday evening's meal was minimal, leftovers from the previous week. However, Easter baskets were prepared for the children, and, while they were working, everyone enjoyed snacking on the sweet treats.

Easter Sunday began with several shifts for breakfast. Marcella's daughters, her grandson, and Anne's son ate their meal of ham, waffles, eggs, and coffee. An hour later the same meal was prepared for and eaten by Marcella's brother, Leo, and his family.

In the afternoon, Marcella, two of her daughters, and her grandson visited Marcella's former mother-in-law and a friend. They had tea and cake. A friend of Marcella's, whose Easter dinner had been catered, gave Marcella a sweet cheese pie with citron that her family did not like.

Nine people were invited for Easter dinner. Roxanne's fiancé and his father brought wine. One of the researchers (with her family) brought chocolate-covered strawberries. One of Marcella's daughters, Jeannette, donated a bottle of homemade wine. The Easter meal consisted of three courses. The first was ravioli, salad, and bread and butter. It was followed by a roast turkey with Italian meat and American bread stuffings, peas and carrots, and wine. Desserts included Anne's rice pudding (she was not present at the meal), chocolate strawberries, *pittalatte*, citron cheese pie (given to Marcella earlier that day), two poundcakes shaped like Easter eggs (given by a friend who works at a local bakery), and the Easter baskets. Later in the evening, Marcella's sister sent over a large pan of lasagna with her son. (It was estimated that the original batch of lasagna had weighed more than ten pounds.)

Marcella distributed leftovers to everyone as they went home. The rest of the food would be redistributed and transformed into various meals during the coming week. In addition, each of the women would send, bring, or exchange her version of the holiday specialties with her family and friends.

The food and eating activities described for this holiday period were intense; ordinarily, such activities and exchanges might take place over two weeks rather than one. However, though the timing was compressed, the varieties of food exchange during this period are representative of patterns of reciprocity in this community.

Patterns of Exchange: The Coopers

Anne's exchange activities are much more limited than Marcella's. Although she is a member of the same mid-life generational cohort, she has circumscribed her sphere of interaction, focusing on family and a few friends. (See Figure 7.2 for a diagram of relationships among participants.) She regularly engages in the exchange of hospitality (meals, prepared foods, and visiting) with her son's family, her two sisters, and the Fiore family. During the week described here, Anne and Marcella shared some meals at restaurants and prepared an elaborate Sunday dinner together. However, even within this circumscribed sphere, exchange activities are significant. Anne's social ties (demonstrated through food exchange) are confined to family (two sisters and her son and his family) and a few

Anne

Natal family

Sisters

Jane   Margaret (Sam)

Conjugal family

Son	*Daughter*	*Son*
Bobby (Mary)	Susan (John)	Jerry
Debbie		

Intimate friendship network

Louise   Marcella
               Andrea   Roxanne

F I G U R E 7.2
Major Participants in Exchange Activities: Relationship to Anne

friends (Marcella and Louise). Here, we see how differing ability and reputation as a traditional cook and a differing number of social ties, despite a comparable stage in the domestic cycle, produce sharp contrasts in food exchange activity.

On Sunday, Susan (Anne's daughter), Marcella's daughter Andrea, and one of their mutual friends went shopping together and ate at the local pizza parlor. During the afternoon, Anne attended a baby shower at the home of her cousin in honor of her cousin's daughter-in-law. The buffet meal included meatballs in gravy, hot roast beef for sandwiches, potato salad, macaroni salad, cold cuts, rolls, vodka punch, two kinds of cake, pizzelles (which Anne's sister Jane had baked), and coffee and tea. Anne's daughter-in-law Mary invited Anne, her daughter Susan, and one of the researchers to dinner that evening. She served roast chicken, mashed potatoes, vegetables, and lobster tails. The latter were brought by Susan for her brother; they were the remains of a meal she and her boyfriend, John, had eaten the previous evening. Dessert consisted of several kinds of cake, one of which was the top layer of the wedding cake from Mary and her husband's reception in Maryton; it had been frozen for two years.

There was a blizzard on Monday. The roads were not plowed and Anne did not go to work. One of the employees of the Cooper business came to get Susan to take her to work. He ate breakfast with Anne and her daughter. Anne prepared cheese steaks for dinner. The weather disrupted her usual pattern, which was to serve filet mignon for Monday's dinner. Later on, her son Jerry returned from a trip to Florida, bringing citrus fruits and pecans. Anne made him a cheese steak as well.

On Wednesday, Anne served "eggs in gravy" (eggs simmered in tomato sauce) for lunch. This was a favorite dish that her mother always made. During the afternoon, Anne's sister Margaret and her husband, Sam (Bob Cooper Sr.'s brother) dropped by for coffee. That evening, pastina beef soup was combined with grilled-cheese sandwiches for dinner (served to her daughter, one of the researchers, and her son). Anne "saved a platter" for Jerry, as she often did when he worked late, keeping it warm in the oven.

Thursday evening's dinner menu was constructed in response to Susan's request for *gnocchis*, her favorite kind of macaroni. Plans for Sunday's big meal were discussed; Marcella would make a pecan pie (with pecans brought by Jerry from Florida) and help in the preparation of *pastacina* (an elaborate baked macaroni dish) and *brasciole* (rolled flank steak stuffed with hard-boiled eggs and cheese). Both dishes were family favorites, and the meal would take two days to prepare.

On Friday, Anne and one of the researchers did a weekly shopping and also bought specific foods for Sunday's dinner. That evening, Anne, Marcella, and the two researchers went out to dinner.

The two women began to cook on Saturday afternoon, preparing the components of Sunday's festive meal: gravy, meatballs, *brasciole*, and rice pudding. Marcella brought an assortment of pastries for a treat while they worked. At each step of the preparation process, they compared cooking styles: "I usually do it this way," said Marcella; "I'll do it my way," Anne sang in reply. Anne did make her gravy somewhat differently than usual, using "bones" (pig knuckles) for a better flavor. This was to be kept secret from her children, who would not eat the gravy if they knew. Andrea and Susan arrived in time to eat meatballs just out of the oven, which everyone loved. Anne gave Marcella a pineapple cheesecake that no one in her family liked. Marcella took it home for her daughter Roxanne.

Twelve people were invited to Sunday dinner: Anne's son Bobby and his family, Marcella and Andrea, Susan's boyfriend, and both researchers (plus Theophano's husband and child). Anne's daughter-in-law Mary arrived during the afternoon to help with last-minute preparations. As she put together the *pastacina* (layers of macaroni, gravy, mozzarella cheese, pepperoni, hard boiled eggs, ham, and grated cheese), Anne worried about how it would taste— "It better come stringy," she said. Mary recalled how Anne had sent food to Bobby at college: frozen gravy, meatballs, and *pastacina*. Bobby, Jerry, and their father snacked on meatballs and sausage before dinner. While they were sitting at the kitchen table, Marcella and Andrea walked in the door with three pecan pies and one pie without pecans for Susan. Anne asked Marcella to prepare the salad for dinner. Anne and Marcella did not sit down to eat until everyone was served. They were "up and down" for extra gravy and bread and for forgotten items. Marcella ate the pig knuckles in the kitchen in order to hide them from the Cooper children. Anne's sons cleared the table in preparation for coffee and dessert, which they served. This was unusual, and Andrea commented "You just want your dessert without waiting." After everything was cleaned up, the older generation sat in the kitchen and talked about their early lives in the immigrant neighborhoods of the community. Anne's son Bobby telephoned to remind his mother to save him some *pastacina* that he had forgotten to take home.

Marcella's pivotal position in the network is continually defined by the frequency and sheer volume of the exchange she commands, either through giving or receiving. In fact, the week we have described in her home does not include shared shopping activity, daily visitors to her office, or the frequent lunch and dinner guests during an ordinary week. In contrast, Anne's position is reflected in the narrower range of reciprocity that surrounds her. In addition, the *kinds* of items exchanged reveal the position of the women we have described. Marcella's status is enhanced by her knowledge of traditional cooking, a skill not widely shared by the community. She most often trades in these exotica and contributes to innovation and variation in the food system. She adapts, adopts, and invents new recipes, always employing a wide variety of items, both familiar and exotic, in her repertory. Anne is not as confident in the domain of traditional cooking and limits her preparation of "Italian" foods. She exchanges food primarily with her children and is limited to a few dishes, primarily baked goods. Despite this limitation, food exchange is as vital a component of Anne's interaction as it is of Marcella's.

THE FORMS, PRINCIPLES, AND TIMING OF RECIPROCITY

The forms of exchange are multiple. They include the exchange of hospitality (inviting guests for meals, eating at someone else's home); sharing nonmealtime eating activities (planned or spontaneous); exchanging raw or cooked foods; payment for services with specialties or favorite foods (these are also used as gifts); and cooperative preparation of family dinners, holiday meals, and food for other events. This latter category involves the pooling of time, money, and foodstuffs, with subsequent redistribution of prepared foods as gifts or leftovers. The flow of reciprocity is also influenced by the food event and by the formats selected to celebrate these occasions. The formats involve different kinds of cooperation and different contributions.

Exchange items are drawn largely from the Italian repertory of the system. The ability of a "gravy" or "one-pot" meal to accommodate a larger group than the immediate family, together with the more celebratory nature of these meal formats, often generates larger attendance lists. The week preceding Easter in Marcella's home is a good example of cooperative labor and extended family and friendship meals. Such meals are also divisible and portable in ways that the American platter format is not. This is not to say that guests are not invited to share platter meals or that the whole-meat alternative is not selected for extended family Sunday or holiday dinners: Many platter meals are responsive to guests' or family members' known likes or particular requests. However, a platter meal is not as likely to be sent to another home as a gift, in repayment for service, and the like, as would be portions of "gravy" or "one-pot" meals. Nor will women of several households cooperatively prepare such a meal.

Desserts (homemade and purchased) are also frequent exchange items. In this case, foods from the American tradition are more frequently exchanged. Italian sweets (cookies, breads, puddings, and pies) are associated with particular periods or occasions and limited to them. For example, during the Christmas season a variety of baked goods (*crustellis*, chocolate pepper cookies, *biscotti*, several versions of *taralles*) are prepared. Several women will share the cost and labor of preparation and distribute the specialties to members of their families and to friends. Other holidays, such as Easter and festive occasions (showers, weddings) are also associated with particular baked goods.

Principles

Reciprocity is governed by principles of rank and distance; thus, the most critical condition for the flow of exchange is the relationship among the participants. Symmetrical relationships are defined as equal relationships between peers and generational cohorts. Asymmetrical relationships include those in which generational or status differences are present, that is, those based on marriage, maternity, or occupational status. High intimacy indicates relationships among immediate and extended family members in addition to members of the friendship network who interact frequently. Low intimacy refers to relationships among distant kin, workmates, and less frequently seen friends. When intimacy and symmetry are both present in a relationship, greater demands are placed on the individuals to exchange. At the same time there is flexibility in the amount of time permitted for reciprocity to occur.

Temporal Sequencing

Reciprocity is a continuum; the instances of exchange range from immediate repayment to reciprocity over a longer period. Almost all social interaction is accompanied by some form of food, and frequent social interaction engenders frequent occasions for exchange.

The ongoing social life of this community is punctuated by an annual cycle of recurrent, predictable events such as birthdays, anniversaries, calendrical holidays, association and club meetings, and special family dinners. On the other hand, weddings, confirmations, and graduations are examples of the milestone occasions generated by the life cycle, which happen only once in the life of an individual.

Reciprocity may be immediate or of long duration; its form may be labor, money, or goods. The differentiating principle for the form and timing of exchange is the occasion itself.

For recurrent occasions, the repayment may occur immediately or at a later time. Family dinners are occasions that most often generate immediate exchange. However, intimate peers are not required to fulfill this obligation immediately, as it is expected that reciprocity will occur in the long run because of the nature of the relationship. Milestone events engender a similar pattern for intimate peers. Repayment may occur immediately, but it is more likely to be of longer duration. However, for such infrequent and high feasts as weddings, repayment is neither appropriate nor expected except in the form of labor or the donation of baked goods, such as cookies. Daughters, who are generationally different but close, are not expected to reciprocate for recurrent occasions unless they wish to do so. For both kinds of events, this group is expected to fulfill their obligations at some future time. Less intimate peers are repaid or must fulfill their obligations for repayment immediately or soon after receipt of a gift for recurrent events. They are under the same obligations as asymmetrical nonintimates for these occasions. Milestone events exhibit another pattern; nonintimate peers are expected to fulfill obligations at some future time, while there are no expectations for those younger, older, or of lesser status. Variability in the pattern of food exchange is shaped by temporal sequencing and frequency, form of ex-

T A B L E 7.3
Expectations for Reciprocity

Category of Relationship	Category of Occasion	
	Recurrent	Milestone
High intimacy		
symmetrical	immediate	immediate
	----------▶	----------▶
	long duration	long duration
asymmetrical	no expectation	long duration
Low intimacy		
symmetrical	immediate	long duration
asymmetrical	immediate	no expectation

Note:
Intimate—immediate/extended family
         friendship network (frequent contact)
Distant—workmates, friendship network (infrequent contact)

Symmetrical—peers/members of the same generational cohort
Asymmetrical—generational differences
              status differences

change, category of occasion, and the nature of the relationship between the participants (see Table 7.3).

CONCLUSION

We have discussed the role of food exchange in symbolizing and constituting social relationships in several households. In the Maryton study, we identified various influences in the exchange process that have to do with household characteristics. Generational cohort is a pivotal feature. We examined in detail the exchange activities of a group of women who have spent their lives in Maryton (see Curtis 1983). They demonstrate their lifelong and multiple social ties through continual interaction, accompanied by the sharing and exchanging of food. Although the mid-life group is most active in the exchange system, and is its anchor, younger families participate as well, particularly the daughters of the mid-life cohort. Stage in the domestic cycle does influence the scope of exchange activities, however. Responsibilities for young and school-aged children can limit a woman's involvement in a female friendship network, narrowing her exchange sphere to conjugal and natal family members.

As we have indicated, exchange activities are responsive as well to the number of a woman's social ties and to her position in the community. Related to these is a woman's reputation as a cook, which reflects not only her culinary abilities but generational cohort and status as well.

Over time, households change developmentally, as do the women. The consequent reorganization of personnel engenders a constantly widening and narrowing unit. If we consider food exchange in all its forms—hospitality (inviting guests for meals, eating at someone else's home); sharing nonmealtime eating activities; exchanging raw or cooked foods; paying for services with special foods; and cooperatively preparing family dinners, holiday meals, and the like—then the household unit shifts in structure with nearly every eating event and related activity.

We would like to discuss briefly the implication of food exchange for consumption, allocation, and expenditure. During the two months we spent in Marcella's household, guests were present for meals or other food events on more than a hundred occasions. In addition to her own family (and one researcher), Marcella frequently fed ten extra people. Food (either raw or prepared) was exchanged in this network almost every day, for a total of fifty-eight exchange occurrences. The exchanges included shared cost, prepared foods, raw items, and leftovers. Most often, Marcella distributed prepared foods (main courses for meals) and received raw foodstuffs or desserts. Marcella spent just over $200.00 on food in each month. (This figure includes her contribution to holiday preparations.) Despite being based on 1979 prices, which were even then beginning to rise, this expenditure is very low for the number of people who were being provisioned.

During our month in the Cooper home, Anne regularly prepared meals for five family members and one researcher. She participated in sixteen exchange occurrences and had guests for thirty food events, ranging from "coffee" to Sunday dinner. She also spent just over $200.00 on food. Thus, even restricted exchange activity is significant.

Exchange, therefore, in addition to representing social links and differences, constitutes a significant means of provisioning households. Shopping, distributing leftovers, and preparing large quantities of food are part of the system of exchange and are often important means for provisioning other households. Participation in such a cooperative network of exchange has implications for social and nutritional policy concerns. Most social and medical programs are based on a model that identifies the individual or the family as the locus of decision making about food and health. Here, as for other groups in variable economic situations (Rapp 1978; Stack 1974; Lamphere 1974), integration in social networks has been shown to be significant in household decision making and provisioning.

The system of food exchange also has consequences for innovation, variation, and conservatism in the diet.[3] Holidays are occasions when the preparation of traditional items can reinforce conservatism in the sense of continuity over time. However, formats for holidays are far from rigid, and the process of menu negotiation produces variation from family to family and from year to year, as well as innovations in meal formats and the preparation of special foods. Innovation in the ordinary cycle may be accomplished through the introduction of a network member's specialty into regular menu planning and through the sharing of different preparation techniques and preferences for particular ingredients. The exchange of prepared foods, recipes, and cyclical specialties also influences the variation in household patterns of food consumption.

We have discussed some of the characteristics that shape food exchange in Maryton. Through the food system, women express and maintain their social positions in the community: They are bound by relationships of mutual exchange. Exchanging food in Maryton is a token of social bonding and integral to all social interaction.

NOTES

Acknowledgments: Portions of this research were funded by National Science Foundation through a grant to Temple University. We would like to thank David Feingold and Karen Kerner for their initial collaboration on this effort. The participant observation phase was supported by the Russell Sage Foundation as part of the Project on Gastronomic Categories, overseen by Mary Douglas. The Italian-American component of the project was directed by Judith Goode. Finally, the work would not have been possible without the generosity of the women of Maryton. Our ongoing interaction contributes to a deeper understanding of the complexity of their responsibility for family and community life.

1. These differences are expanded in Curtis and Theophano 1981.

2. We have found this to be true in Maryton. Other descriptions of Italian-American women firmly eschew this perspective (di Leonardo 1984).

3. We have previously described the comparative nutritional consequences of different components of the diet; the generic category of "gravy" (the Italian portion of the diet) is more nutritionally adequate with respect to vegetable and saturated fat consumption (Goode, Curtis, and Theophano 1984).

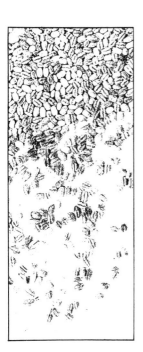

CHAPTER 8

From Generation to Generation: Resources, Experience, and Orientation in the Dietary Patterns of Selected Urban American Households

Anne Sharman

In choosing questions to ask and suggesting an approach for analyzing her material, Anne Sharman draws particularly on recent developments in the analysis of food and culture and on marxist and other analyses of social inequality and social stratification. Her aim is to find a way of relating the complexities of people's position and experience in a system of social stratification to variability, continuity, and change in their domestic organization and dietary practices.

She worked with African Americans, who, when she started her research, had low incomes and were eligible for the Special Supplemental Food Program for Women, Infants, and Children (WIC). Many of the people, however, experienced substantial fluctuations in income, and their circumstances were correspondingly changeable. They also showed considerable variation in their residential, educational, and occupational histories; the histories of their natal families; and their current relationships, activities, and sources of income. They were affiliated with a variety of Protestant churches and with Muslim temples, recognized a number of different general food systems, and had varied dietary practices.

To analyze the complexities of this situation Sharman needs a framework that will emphasize processes giving rise to outcomes, that can take into account larger-scale organization, and that can incorporate events over a longer period than is generally covered in analyses. She also seeks an approach that will give people an active voice in describing events, their own orientations, and their attempts to shape the conditions of their existence. The analysis of life histories seems to present the possibility of such a framework and approach.

Analysis of life histories represents a new departure in nutritional anthropology, another method of looking at the interrelationships between factors affecting dietary practices. It opens up new possibilities for examining the transmission of dietary practices from one generation to the next and for studying the process of socialization as it takes place throughout people's lives. Finally, in allowing individuals to tell their story it is an approach that can bring new understanding of people's long- and short-term goals, strategies, and choices and the salience of food and diet in their lives.

General patterns of continuity and change in the diets of culturally defined groups have been quite widely studied. Little work has been done, however, on the processes by which dietary practices are transmitted from one generation to the next (Shultz and Theophano 1984). Occasional studies that have focused on the transmission of food behaviors and preferences using statistical analysis have not been able to isolate factors giving rise to observed differences and similarities between members of successive generations (Kolasa 1974). This chapter suggests, through the presentation of case studies, how an analysis of people's life histories can contribute to an understanding of the development of their dietary practices and of the processes underlying continuity, change, and variability within and between generations.

The focus is on five households. Three of them are those of sisters who grew up together, one is that of a woman related to them by marriage (see Figure 8.1) and the fifth household is that of the parents of the three sisters.[1] These case studies indicate the importance of individual life histories by showing the variation that has developed among the households of people with very similar backgrounds.[2] Presentation of detailed information on the life histories of a few people makes it possible to illustrate the complexity of the interrelations among the many factors that bear on people's dietary patterns, as well as the importance of analyzing not just outcomes but also processes giving rise to outcomes. "In addition to their analytical power . . . life histories also possess a synthetic power" (Bertaux and Kohli 1984, 215).

POPULATION AND SETTING

The data used in this paper were collected as part of a study in a section of a large northeastern city. The study explored the relationship between dietary choices and allocation of resources within households, with particular attention to the effect of low incomes and the impact of the Special Supplemental Food Program for Women, Infants, and Children (WIC) (see Sharman 1984). To facilitate study of factors affecting choices within households, where

July 1978

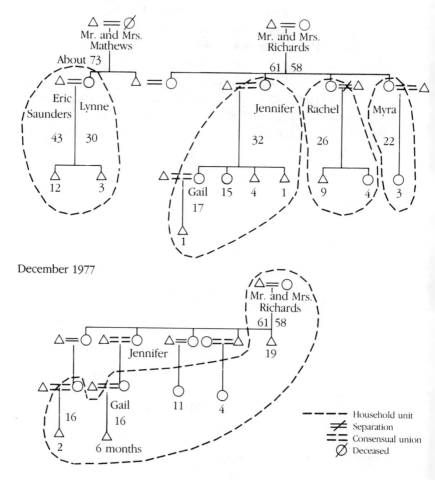

Note: All names are pseudonyms. Gail moved from Mr. and Mrs. Richards's to her mother's house between December 1977 and July 1978.

F I G U R E 8.1

Relationships Between, and Composition of, Case-Study Households, on Date Specified

variations between them would not be linked to major racial/ethnic and income/class differences, people were chosen for the study who belonged to the same racial/ethnic category and had similar incomes. African Americans with low incomes were selected because they were the majority of the clients at a clinic in which I was working as a volunteer on the WIC Program when I started the research. This situation arose because of residential segregation. The clinic was located on the edge of a housing project in which virtually all families with young children were African American.

The population served by the clinic was concentrated in about ten by five major blocks (but was spread over a wider area). This area included a housing project and other low-income housing, both public and private, and was characterized by marked racial and ethnic divisions in some sections. The racial and ethnic composition of the population, however, was usually not the same for more than four or five blocks, and, as the area had been affected greatly by the "urban renaissance," people of different incomes and classes lived in close proximity in some places. Thus it was a very varied district, extending over more than one locally defined neighborhood, and the people in it had access to a variety of shopping facilities. Furthermore, a bus ride or a twenty- to forty-five-minute walk could take inhabitants into different sections of the main shopping area of the city.

DATA COLLECTION

Data collection centered on compiling information for particular case studies. Selection was of women with children under five, but men also actively participated, and data were always collected on women and their young children in the context of a particular household(s). The household was defined as all those people who regularly slept in the same dwelling or spent much of their time there and contributed toward the rent (or had a contribution made on their behalf). Households thus defined were also significant eating and budgeting units, although there were sometimes identifiable subunits within them, their boundaries were often flexible, and they were not exclusive. In the most cases they had close ties of kinship and friendship with other households in the area, which led to frequent movement of goods, services, and people among them. There were often definite differences in dietary patterns between households, and when people changed households they sometimes changed their eating patterns in significant ways.

Initial selection of people was from among those receiving the WIC Program at the clinic where I worked, to which a few others were added. People were divided into three categories on the basis of age: those under twenty, those aged twenty to twenty-nine, and those aged thirty and over. Within each age category people were chosen for a variety of reasons but primarily to represent households and individuals with a range of characteristics as regards relation of children under five to household head, number and ages of children, household composition, marital status, education, employment history, number of relatives in the area, and type of housing. Detailed information was collected for twenty-three case studies. Additional material was obtained for a further seventeen households and through a variety of other contacts.

Most data were gathered periodically from fall 1977 through summer 1980. Information on diet, activity patterns, and income and expenditure was collected for different seasons, together with information on other aspects of people's food habits, economic and social position, domestic relationships, and personal (and in some cases family) histories. Methods of data collection included recorded interviews, record books, informal discussions, observation, participant observation, and the medical records of children. Life history data were mostly obtained through recording open-ended interviews based on an aide-mémoire and by doing genealogies. Relevant aspects of peoples' lives and their perceptions of them were also learned about during participant observation and other social interaction.

CULTURAL CONTEXT

The people with whom I worked refer to different food systems in a very general sense when they describe and justify how they eat.[3]

The food systems identified in this way reflect the historical experience of African Americans, some of their responses to this experience, and the situation of this particular population in a complex and changing urban environment. Thus, people refer to southern food, soul food, Muslim food, and health food; they talk about the things they eat all the time (chicken and rice, for example); they discuss what white people eat and white people's stereotypes and perceptions of what they eat; and they talk about what people with money can afford to eat and what they themselves might like to eat sometimes or more often if they had more money (steak, seafood, food from the health food stores, and so on). Different food systems thus referred to are defined by different criteria—regional, racial/ethnic, religious, income/class, health—and may be perceived as having more than one referent.

Thus, for example, southern food refers to a food system associated not only with a southern heritage but also with a heritage of slavery. Soul food is often seen as deriving from this same heritage and as being typically southern food, but it is also the food African Americans eat, the food they share, savor, and enjoy, the food that unites them and enables them to survive. These different referents can lead members of different income/class and racial/ethnic categories to perceive and categorize the same foods differently. Thus Whitehead (1984) in his study of a southern community reports:

> For example, the lower SES [Socio-Economic Status] black and middle SES white KKPs [Key Kitchen Persons] referred to such pork products as neck bones, "fat back," feet, ears, and tails; chicken necks, feet, giblets, and backs; black-eyed peas, and dried beans as "poor people's food." Lower SES whites and middle SES blacks, however, considered the same items "black people's food." (115)

He also shows that these different views are reflected in patterns of consumption. Furthermore, in other situations it can also be seen that because soul food is the food African Americans eat, it can mean different foods in different contexts. It can be any food that African Americans are eating, it can exclude pork, it can be vegetarian (Burgess 1976; Dengler 1979).

As well as soul food and southern food, other general food

systems also overlap and are interrelated in different ways. This is the case even for southern food and Muslim food, though Muslims reject the southern heritage of poverty and oppression and with it pork and sometimes other components of southern foods, such as black-eyed peas, lima beans, collard greens, sweet potatoes, and corn. These were suggested as foods to be avoided when Elijah Muhammad originally set out dietary prohibitions and recommendations in *How to Eat to Live* (1967, 1972).[4]

There is a continuity that transcends the content of the diet associated with being poor in the south. A recurring theme is the link people feel between the positive aspects of the way their families managed to live their lives in the harsh conditions of the south and the Muslim way of feeding and nurturing their families. What they see as reminiscent of their life in the south is the strong emphasis, in Muslim teaching and Muslim practice, on the importance of family life and of food preparation and cooking in nurturing and caring for family members; on women's role as nurturers; and on doing things the natural, wholesome way, such as breast-feeding babies and cooking meals from scratch. An example of such perceived continuity may be found in the life history and dietary patterns of Lynne, who is a Muslim. This faith's teachings, particularly on the health hazards of pork, also influence numerous people who are not themselves Muslims, as a result of many Christians having close kin and affines (sometimes living in the same household), friends, and neighbors who are Muslim, and as a result of information provided during recruitment drives.

Again, the emphasis on health in Muslim teaching—for example, doing things the natural way, not overeating, and limiting consumption of meat—also links the Muslim movement in some ways with the health food movement. In fact, all these general food systems carry with them ideas of how they are related to the standard American food system. The concept of American food, however, is not usually evoked by people as an explanation or a justification of particular ways of eating (except sometimes in relation to English food when talking to me, since I come from England). Rather, it is a question of recognizing that some of the things they eat are much the same as those that all Americans eat, especially generally used fast foods and prepackaged meals, whereas other foods derive from their own particular heritage. They also refer to, and sometimes cook, dishes that they see as deriving from other cultural traditions, such as Chinese, Hawaiian, and so on. A number of people placed a high value on experimentation and innovation in food preparation.

These different ideas about food and patterns of eating, and the traditions and experiences to which they refer, provide a repertoire from which people select what they will eat. It is a knowledge and an understanding of the repertoire that, to varying degrees and with varying expertise, they share, rather than particular patterns of eating. Opinions are expressed, sometimes forcefully, about how women cater for their households, but there is also accepted flexibility in ways of doing things. The repertoire that people share can in part be presented through some general meal formats characteristic of breakfast, lunch, and dinner in the population (see Table 8.1). Tables 8.2 and 8.3 list the choices made for breakfast and dinner by the five case study households for a week in the month indicated during 1977 and 1978. Breakfasts include what might be described as brunches; dinner means the main meal of the day, whether it is eaten in the afternoon or the evening. Lunches are not included because they are always quick meals, and variations are less significant in relation to the discussion in this chapter. Data included in Tables 8.2 and 8.3 were collected using record books, but discussion of the data, which follows brief presentation of the life histories of the heads of the households (using the ethnographic present), is also informed by data collected at other times, using interviews, record books, and interaction with members of the households.

LIFE HISTORIES

Individual life histories varied considerably among the people with whom I worked. Households being studied included ones headed by people who migrated from the south forty or more years ago, who came north within the last five years, who grew up in the rural northeast, who had lived all their lives in the urban northeast, and

who were born and raised in the section of the city where I
worked. The education of adult household members ranged from
seven years to two people with university degrees. The majority had
completed some years of high school but had not graduated, while
some teenage mothers were still at school. During the course of the
study a number of people were trying to obtain a high school diploma or some other form of training, and two women attended
the local community college, eventually going on to obtain their
B.A. degrees elsewhere.

Occupations during the time I was doing the study, and occupational histories, also varied. Jobs included a wide range of often
short-term, part-time or seasonal, low-paid, unskilled, and semi-
skilled manual and service work, as well as teaching (a teacher laid
off through no fault of her own and a teachers' aide) and community work (a graduate looking for a job, who subsequently found
one). Some people unable to obtain paid employment also volun-
teered their services to institutions unwilling or unable to pay
them, such as the schools their children attended. Some people in
the population were upwardly mobile and have obtained full-time
employment, which has enabled them to become independent of
any form of government assistance. Others were downwardly mobile and, though dependent on government assistance when I was
working with them, had previously had reliable, full-time jobs and
had lived in better circumstances. Finally, people belonged to a
wide variety of Protestant churches, including Lutheran, Baptist, and
Jehovah's Witnesses, and to Muslim temples. Few attended Catholic
churches, although some sent their children to Catholic schools
when they could find the money to do so.

Both Mr. and Mrs. Richards and Mr. and Mrs. Mathews (Figure
8.1) were born and grew up in the same locality in South Carolina,
where they were all members of the Baptist church. They left the
area, where they worked as landless farm laborers, some forty years
ago, and finally settled in the same part of the northeastern city
where they live now. Lynne, Jennifer, Rachel, and Myra were all
born in the city and have lived in roughly the same area for most of
their lives; all four have a network of close kin and affines there,
together with other relatives and friends and acquaintances. Eric,

also raised in the city, grew up an orphan and only met his brothers and sisters again later in life. When I was working with them they all lived in a housing project, except Mr. Mathews, who lived in a rented accommodation nearby. Eric did not finish high school. Lynne, Jennifer, Rachel, and Myra all left school between the tenth and twelfth grades, as did Jennifer's daughter Gail, and none of them felt that she learned much about food and nutrition at school. Although the duration of the employment of the heads of the households varied, it was generally in low-paid unskilled and semi-skilled manual and service work. Mr. and Mrs. Richards, Jennifer, Rachel, and Myra are all still Baptist; Eric is Muslim; and Lynne converted from Baptist to Muslim in the early 1970s.

Lynne

Lynne was the youngest of seven children and so, she says, stayed close to her mother for a long time. She was always in the kitchen with her and learned to cook early. Her mother was known as a real southern cook, both in the sense of cooking very palatable food from scratch and in the sense that she cooked foodstuffs associated with life in the south. Lynne describes, however, how her mother's repertoire of recipes was expanded in the city; how, for example, she learned ways of cooking tripe and spaghetti sauce from an Italian-American neighbor, for whom her daughter used to run errands. Lynne is said to be the best cook among her siblings, although she is the only Muslim in her immediate family, is described as a southern cook, is the one whose cooking her father will eat most willingly, and is the one to whom her sisters turn for help. When she became a Muslim she learned new methods of cooking at the temple; now, when she prepares dishes traditionally seasoned with pork she makes substitutions, as in the record week, when she cooked black-eyed peas for dinner and seasoned them with smoked turkey wings rather than with ham hocks. She does not, however, currently follow all the prohibitions and recommendations set out by Elijah Muhammad and ate lima beans (though green limas) and sweet potatoes, as well as black-eyed peas, in the same week.

The importance of dietary practices in Muslim teaching has re-inforced a knowledge of, and interest in, nutrition that Lynne ob-tained from her employment over the years. After she left school in the twelfth grade, she worked in a hospital as a dietitians' aide (a job obtained for her by her mother) and since then has worked in various capacities as a nurses' aide, when the hours, job oppor-tunities, and her health permit (she, her husband, and her two sons are all asthmatic), with occasional periods in non-health-related jobs. Her husband has worked seasonally as a construction worker and as a presser in a dry cleaners. Because of their employment, Lynne and Eric's overall regular income is higher than that of the other households, and they are only intermittently eligible for Aid to Families with Dependent Children (AFDC) and food stamps. But the jobs they have are often low-paid and insecure, so that their higher income is to some extent offset by its unreliability. In sum-mer 1978 she was not employed, but her husband was.

If only one of them is employed, they need, and often have to struggle to obtain, food stamps and sometimes supplementary AFDC payments. Periodically, they have emergency periods when neither of them is employed and no government assistance is re-ceived. At such times they are hard pressed to maintain their eating patterns and have to rely on daily help in the form of small amounts of money and goods from their immediate family (Eric's sisters and brothers; Lynne's sister and father) and must reluctantly withdraw from savings. Lynne and Eric are constantly planning ways to leave the project and buy a house. When this has been achieved, Lynne plans to get her high school diploma or GED (high school diploma equivalent) and train as a nurse.

Jennifer

Jennifer is the second of eight children; in her natal family it seems to have been the older daughters who learned to cook and who remain the most skilled. By the time Rachel and Myra were growing up, Rachel says, there were older girls to help and her mother was tired of teaching her daughters to cook. Rachel and Myra are the fifth and seventh children, respectively, and the last two girls. Mrs. Richards is again described as a good southern cook and is generous and tough in providing for her household. Of her children, Jennifer seems to be regarded as the best cook, but her situation is quite different from that of Lynne in her natal family, and her skill is less clear in her current dietary patterns.

Jennifer left school at fifteen when she became pregnant, but her basic literacy and math skills are at least equal to those of the others. She worked in a number of different low-paid jobs, none of them nutrition or health related, after her child was old enough to be looked after by her mother. When she was approximately twenty-four, she moved out of her parents' house into an apartment in the housing project and at about that time started working full-time as a presser at the cleaners where her eldest sister works. She stopped full-time work when her oldest son was born, but still works for short periods during holiday seasons when regular employees are away. With two small children of her own, her teenage daughters, and one grandchild (with another on the way), as well as little support apart from that of her immediate family, it is difficult for Jennifer to envisage many opportunities for herself, and her health is poor. She concentrates on improving her household's living conditions (she moved from an apartment to a house in the project) and on the task of budgeting her resources and getting together what her household needs. Of the four households, hers is the one with the sparsest resources. In juggling her finances she has fallen behind in her rent; she does not have a phone, but uses that of her parents; she uses her parents' or her sisters' irons; and she has a minimum of furniture.

Rachel

Rachel's orientation and disposition are very different from those of Jennifer, and in some ways from those of Lynne too, although she and Lynne share hope and drive in their goals for themselves and their children. Rachel did not learn to cook at home; when she got married at the age of eighteen, her husband helped her and she also learned from his mother and sister. Even now she does not really like to cook, never bakes from scratch, and seeks help from her mother sometimes for more elaborate cooking.

Before her son was born, Rachel worked for a short while in a clothes factory; after that, she was married, had her daughter, and did not work again until about three years ago, when she worked as a parent–scholar at her children's school. She has, however, been going to various schools to get her GED; has tried for other jobs; and is very active at her children's school and at her Baptist church. She is vice-chairperson of the PTA at school and, among other things, was chairperson of the committee to raise money for women's day at the church.

What follows is an example of a weekday for her in September 1978, when the schools were in session. She got up at 7:15, washed and dressed her daughter, and gave the children breakfast. The children left the house about 8:15, her son to school and her daughter to her mother's house. She studied for a short time, since she herself was attending school, but was interrupted by her sister coming by to borrow bleach. She then tried to take a bath, but the phone kept ringing, so she gave up. Then I came by, and a friend of her sister's arrived at the same time. After that she again tried to study and finally went out to school about 12:15; she was back by 3:00. The children were already out of school and she went by her mother's house to check on them. Her son was out selling school candy, and her daughter was playing outside. She left them doing these things and went up to her apartment. She had hardly got in when her sister came by and persuaded her to accompany her to compare supermarket prices. She returned from that outing about 5:30. She quickly fixed her daughter's dinner (her son was still out), and then she and her daughter went to choir practice. She ate some soup when she got back at 9:00. Her son was at her parents', and he ate and slept there. She and her daughter slept at her house.

Of Jennifer, Myra, and herself, Rachel is the one most able to meet her expenses, while, at the same time, helping other family members and investing in such items as a washing machine, which neither her sisters nor Lynne have. And, although her regular income is lower than Lynne's, it is more reliable, and she is helped out by gifts from other people in her social network. Nevertheless, perhaps because of the help she gives others, budgeting is always a struggle, and an apparently small extra expense can sometimes make her seriously short of money. Thus, in the week she organized an expedition to the skating rink for the church, she had to pay an extra $15 for a ticket she had been unable to sell; that expenditure made her so short of money that she had to walk some distance to school for most of the week.

Myra

Myra is the seventh child in the Richards family and the youngest girl. She only moved from her parents' home about two years ago, and she is in no hurry to establish total independence. As with Rachel, Myra never really learned to cook in her natal home and does not enjoy cooking. Jennifer and another sister are helping her to learn, and she sometimes calls her mother for advice, but she still does not cook much herself.

Myra dropped out of school in the eleventh grade and went to look after the children of a sister who lives in another part of the city and works for the Internal Revenue Service. This sister has encouraged her to go to school to get her GED. She has gone for short periods but each time has dropped out, although she still plans to finish the program. Myra has also looked for jobs; she worked for short periods some four years ago at low-paid jobs that were not nutrition or health related, but then she had her daughter and has not been able to find any work since. Although, of course, her situation puts severe limits on what she can do, it seems to be relatively easy for her to manage within these restrictions. She has only one child to look after, is in some ways still in the process of moving out of her natal home and only partially caters for herself, has many siblings with whom she can exchange assistance, and receives gifts for her child from her child's father.

DIET

How, then, do the life histories and the resulting circumstances of Mr. and Mrs. Richards, Lynne and Eric, Jennifer, Rachel, and Myra affect the routine diets of their households, particularly during the week for which data are presented in Tables 8.2 and 8.3. In discussing this question I will look especially at the degree of elaboration and variety in the breakfast and dinner formats they used and also at the content of meals (the kinds of vegetables, meats, and so on, used and the cooking methods) and at some aspects of the general pattern found during the week. "Elaboration" means the length of time required for preparation, the number of ingredients used in dishes prepared, and the number of components of the meal. "Variety" is the extent to which different formats, or different foods for the same formats, were used during the week.

At breakfast and dinner a major distinction is between quick, easy-to-prepare meals and those involving lengthier preparation, although there is clearly a continuum between the two. In most cases there is a combination on weekdays of relatively quick and relatively slow meal formats, at least for dinner, though in some households entirely quick meals are prepared and in others more elaborate meals are prepared most of the time. Another weekday dinner combination, which has been described for African Americans of southern rural origin (Jerome 1980), that of "boiling" and "frying" days, is also found in some households; but in most of them, "frying" days are combined in the week with various quick meals and pasta-based meals. Saturdays are variable, and Sunday dinner is generally a relatively elaborate meal characterized by frying and by roasting or baking. At dinner especially, the content of meals often indicates a particular tradition or a particular focus in people's eating habits, though a cooked breakfast, including cooked cereal and meat, is sometimes associated with the South.

People in the case study households did not necessarily eat the same thing, so the importance of subunits within these households is also discussed. These subunits are distinguished on the basis of people preparing food separately (Jennifer and her daughters) or eating markedly different foods (Rachel and her children), but not on the basis of whether or not people eat at the same time, since such behavior does not define in this population whether or not a meal is shared (Shack 1976).

Mr. and Mrs. Richards

In many respects this household is different from all of the others, although they share similar living conditions and their resources, taking into account household size, are almost as limited as Jennifer's. They belong to an older generation with direct experience of very harsh conditions in the south, of migrating and of making their way in the northeastern city where they now live. They head a large, complex, and flexible household, which forms a center for their many descendants, most of whom still live in the area.

Mrs. Richards generally cooks two relatively elaborate meals a day, breakfast (sometimes mid morning) and dinner, except on Sundays, when she and others attend church and they return to eat dinner early in the afternoon. Mrs. Richards is the only one who seems consistently to use both a traditional southern combination of "boiling" and "frying" days and a contemporary combination of relatively quick and relatively slow meals. She is also the only one who served a variety of a classic southern one-pot meal in the record week, namely, collard greens seasoned with salt pork and served with corn bread. Dinner is almost always (with one exception in the record week) a family meal in this house, in which everyone (except sometimes one of her granddaughters and great-grandsons, who slept at another house during the period) eats what Mrs. Richards provides, though not necessarily at the same time. She sometimes provides quick meals at the children's request or for her own convenience, but she also regularly produces more elaborate meals, though their form may be affected by her limited resources. She also always cooks elaborate breakfasts, but they are not family meals in the sense that dinners are. She cooks breakfast meats primarily for her husband, and sometimes for her son; she also usually eats them herself. Others may share if they are awake, or they may prepare breakfast for themselves if they want to eat before or after she has cooked.

Myra

Myra's small household, consisting only of herself and her daughter, is still particularly close to that of her parents. Thus, for example, during the record week she or her daughter ate dinner at her parents' house four times, once when Myra took a can of spaghetti and heated it herself. She and her daughter also eat frequently at her sisters', and sometimes at the houses of other relatives and friends in the area. Nevertheless, she distinguishes her dietary patterns from those of her parents. When she lived with them, she says, she ate what her mother cooked, but now she no longer eats things she does not like, such as beans, chitterlings (small intestines of pigs), greens, and liver, although she may on occasion prepare them for her boyfriend or her daughter.

Within her own household, Myra eats less frequently (and often differently) than her daughter. She herself is dieting and sometimes barely eats one meal a day, going without or snacking at people's houses, so that she can eat with a clear conscience in the evening, when she gets "the munchies." Her daughter often eats a quick breakfast of cold cereal, but on three occasions in the record week Myra prepared pancakes for her. For dinner she seldom makes meals from scratch, generally using relatively quick, already prepared foods, but she does provide variety in those meals she prepares and often uses meat or fish, starch, and vegetable.

Rachel

Like Myra, Rachel eats differently and more infrequently than her children. In the week for which data are presented, they all ate the same foods only three times for dinner. Rachel often eats only one meal (or one snack) a day and drinks water, juice, and tea at other times. In fact, her mother, who feels she is trying to become too thin, and others were concerned at the severity of her dieting. Later, she did start eating more often in the day, though with care, and usually consuming salads and broiled fish and meat. The meals she prepares for her children show little variety or elaboration. During the record week there was a simple and totally standardized breakfast of sugared cereals and milk (varied with grapes one day) and usually a little-elaborated dinner, generally quick and without vegetables, even when requiring lengthier preparation.

The form and content of these meals seems to reflect lack of time and dislike of cooking, rather than the absence of money, although she does suffer serious shortages at times. When Rachel is short of money for food, she says, she does not make major cuts in what she buys, but she is aware of prices and finds herself putting back some of the items she has selected. During such periods, she says, she finds herself eating a great deal of chicken, a pattern found also in other households. Also, the dietary patterns in her household do not mean that she is unaware of, or uninterested in, good eating practices or unconcerned about good health. She is conscientious in ensuring that her children have good and regular health care, and she leaves them some healthy foods (such as eggs) in the refrigerator to snack on. Her own dieting is for health as well as beauty. What she has not done is to work elaborated eating patterns into her busy schedule, a fact also influenced by what her children will eat most readily.

Jennifer

This household tends to be divided into three (Jennifer and her two young sons, Gail and her son, and Jennifer's younger daughter) and sometimes four (Jennifer and her two young sons eating differently for breakfast) subunits for meals. Breakfasts are often only cold cereals and milk taken out by different people in the household when they are ready, though sometimes someone will prepare a hot cereal or eggs. Jennifer prepares dinner every day for herself and her young sons, and when she is using more elaborated formats she cooks for the whole household and leaves food for her daughters and her grandson to eat when they are ready, as happened four times during the record week, although on one occasion her younger daughter ate differently. When her daughters prepare food separately they only make quick meals. The dinners that Jennifer prepares show greater variety and elaboration than those of her sisters, though less than those of her mother, and hers is the only household (apart from her mother's) in which a stewed or boiled one-pot meal was prepared. She is, however, as already pointed out, the one with the most limited resources, and she sees this and other factors as affecting the dietary patterns of her household.

In talking about what she would like to do, Jennifer has described more elaborations of breakfast menus and more ingredients for such dishes as her stewed beef. She has also remarked on how things have changed in relation to her situation four or five years ago (when she was with her sons' father), when she used to plan and write out her menus each week, have more varied meals, and cook more. Things have changed, she says, because the children have become "funny eaters" and the girls no longer eat at home so much. She says she likes to take food over to her mother's and cook and eat it there with her sons: They like to be with more people and eat better there, and she likes to help her mother cook. Whatever these comments represent, elaboration of her cooking does seem to be limited by her economic and domestic circumstances and possibly by her health.

Lynne

In Lynne and Eric's household, one or both of them may eat differently from their children, and they may eat differently from each other, at breakfast. For dinner, however, there is always a shared family meal, although not all the household members always eat something of everything that is cooked. For dinner particularly the meals Lynne prepares show markedly greater elaboration and variation than those of the other households. Such quick foods as hot dogs are fixed when Lynne is tired (Friday evening in the record week), but ideally they are used only as snacks. Saturday dinner in the record week was also unusual, since the children were away and Lynne and Eric went out. On the other days of the record week Lynne prepared food from scratch each day; had a different meat or form of the same meat every day; and always had meat, vegetable, starch, and sometimes two starches, except on the day she prepared her special sauce for spaghetti and meatballs. As already mentioned, she also prepared such dishes as black-eyed peas and candied sweet potatoes, which are regarded as typically southern and which also, it might be pointed out, take longer to prepare.

The difference in this household's dietary patterns from, for example, Rachel's household, which forms a particularly strong contrast, cannot be attributed primarily to differences in resources of income and time, or in Lynne's and Rachel's orientation and drive toward improving their situation. Nor do they seem to result mainly from Lynne's catering for a household unit of husband and children, and Rachel's catering only for herself and her children. Rather, such differences seem to derive more from the experiences that have led to Lynne and Rachel having different skills in food preparation and to their placing different priorities on cooking more varied and elaborate meals. During emergency periods when Lynne and Eric are particularly short of resources (one of which occurred in September 1978) they do seem to manage to maintain the major outlines of their eating patterns, including the range of meats eaten. But they make adjustments in food purchases and in the details of their food consumption. In September 1978 fruits, desserts, and snacks were cut; quantities (such as those of rice, juices, and sugar) purchased were reduced and made to last as long as quantities purchased previously; and the ingredients of recipes were simplified. In addition, they cut down on other purchases, spent more time and effort (they walked everywhere) combing the area for bargains, and cut down on other activities, doing little visiting and not going to the temple because they felt they had little to contribute.

CONCLUSION

I have used detailed case studies to illustrate the complex ways in which people's life histories affect their dietary practices and to suggest that the particular dietary practices of domestic units at given periods can only be fully understood by looking at the processes by which these patterns have developed, as well as at the current circumstances with which they are associated (see Figure 8.2).

The material presented indicates particularly some of the many direct and indirect ways in which the availability of different resources (for example, income, skill, time) bears on dietary practices in domestic units. Availability and use of resources is in turn related to people's social structural position,[5] the relationships in which

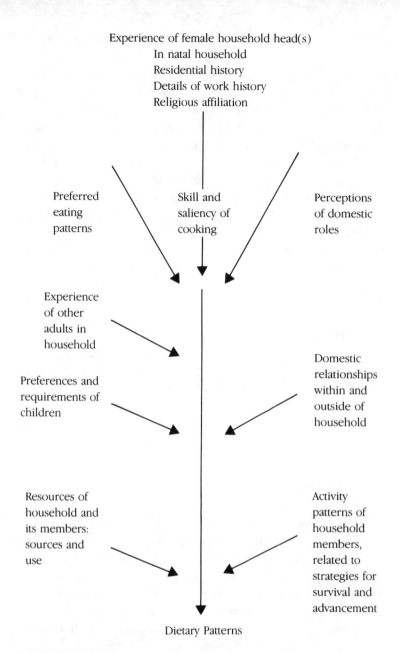

Experience of female household head(s)
In natal household
Residential history
Details of work history
Religious affiliation

Preferred eating patterns

Skill and saliency of cooking

Perceptions of domestic roles

Experience of other adults in household

Preferences and requirements of children

Domestic relationships within and outside of household

Resources of household and its members: sources and use

Activity patterns of household members, related to strategies for survival and advancement

Dietary Patterns

F I G U R E 8.2
Interrelationships Giving Rise to Dietary Patterns Described for
Case-Study Households

they are involved, and the ways in which they perceive and deal with their circumstances. More specifically, in looking at people's life histories it can be seen how their experience in their natal domestic units, and the organization of their own domestic units, is related to their own and to their parents' residential history; their school and subsequent employment history; their responses to their more general social, economic, and political situation, including conversion to Islam;[6] and their orientation in acquiring and using resources for survival and advancement. Food is but one among many resources necessary for survival, good health, and effective performance, and is of varying significance in the lives of different people.

Difficulties inherent in statistical analyses that attempt to isolate and analyze the effects of particular variables on dietary patterns are highlighted by the material presented. It may be possible to identify variables that are likely to be important, such as occupational history, birth order in a person's natal family, Muslim affiliation, low income, and skill in cooking. It is much more difficult to anticipate the effect of these variables in particular contexts, since the context alters their effect and outcomes are the consequences of many cumulative interactions. Interrelations giving rise to dietary patterns can be described, but nothing can be said about how these interrelations will work out, or the dietary patterns they will give rise to in particular domestic units.

Finally, the data I have presented can point to some of the practical limitations of basing nutrition interventions on analysis of outcomes, rather than on analysis of the processes giving rise to outcomes, and of giving inadequate weight to availability of resources and their use. Let me take as an example the use of scalogram analysis of "food complexity" in households and families. Scalogram analysis in this context is used to calculate the level of food complexity in a household, based on what is eaten at a particular point in time. Those using this measure suggest that the scale can be used as an indicator of a household's capacity to process diverse information relating to food, and that a similar capacity will tend to be demonstrated in other areas of the household's life, so that based on this measure nutrition information can be appropriately tailored to fit the household's capacity to process information (Hertzler and Owen 1976).

The data presented in this chapter, however, suggest that it is misleading to base assessments of people's capacity to process dietary information on their dietary practices at a particular time, and that it should not be surprising to find that food complexity and complexity in other areas of people's lives do not coincide. What individuals do at any point depends on many factors. People may have less elaborate and varied diets both because of scarce resources (which also limits culturally valued innovation and experimentation) and because they are focusing on improving their health and their situation through means other than food and nutrition. Furthermore, people with very limited access to resources are frequently involved in processing and acting on very diverse and complex information in their attempts to make ends meet, to maintain an adequate supply of resources, and to improve their situation by, for example, getting better housing and better education for their children. The complex and essentially informal processes in which they are involved, however, are not generally readily visible, nor do they lend themselves to scalogram analysis.

In these circumstances the question for nutrition educators is not how to tailor their message to a limited capacity to process information, although additional nutrition information can be important and helpful to people. It is how to aid people in their attempts to obtain adequate resources (Eide 1982) and how to motivate them to maintain beneficial eating patterns, at the same time as they are trying to improve their situation in other ways essential to good health and performance.

NOTES

Acknowledgments: The research was funded by a Nuffield Foundation Small Grant, National Science Foundation Grant Number BNS 77-14464, and a grant from the National Institutes of Health, Institute of Arthritis,

Metabolism and Digestive Diseases. At the time I was a Senior Research Associate at the Institute for the Study of Human Issues. I wish to thank the members of the institute, together with the many other people (including Anne Okongwu) from whom I received invaluable help and advice during the course of the research, and above all those who with patience, tolerance, and interest accepted my inquiries about their lives. I also wish to thank the individuals whom this chapter is about, and Janet Bujra, Sheila Cosminsky, Suzette Heald, Rosalie Nobles, and Brenda Parish for reading and commenting on earlier versions.

1. Mrs. Mathews died shortly before I met Lynne; Mr. Mathews lived in an apartment on his own.

2. The importance of people's particular experience is also shown in Darden and Darden (1978).

3. Food system as used here includes ideas about food and its availability and selection, ways of cooking, and patterns of preparation and eating. It is not a precise analytical term (in contrast to its usage in Douglas 1984) but a way of denoting an area of discussion.

4. There are different groupings and affiliations among Muslims today. Varying interpretations of, and importance attributed to, the dietary specifications set out by Elijah Muhammad, together with other circumstances, can lead to marked differences in dietary patterns and nutrition between Muslim households.

5. Mullings (1978) has distinguished between two dimensions of ethnicity, the cognitive and the social-structural, the first referring to the content and perception of differences and the second to the way in which these differences are used in the society. It can be deceptive to look only at the cognitive level, and to treat cultural groups and categories as equivalent, when at a social-structural level their situation is very different. She discusses the way in which social-structural constraints have operated for African Americans.

Harrison (1979) demonstrates the fallacy of the idea that there is a distinct "welfare class" of people unwilling or unable to work. He shows that over a period of five years 92 percent of supposedly "ever welfare" households also contained adults who worked at some time. He argues that "any welfare program serves to regulate the supply of low wage labor and to reproduce that labor, and the segment of capital which exploits it. Only if welfare is kept cheap and uncertain can it continue to support capital accumulation" (1).

6. Why some people convert to Islam and others do not (and similarly why some people join other groups, practice innovative behavior, and so on) is another question, but one that again points to the complexity of trying to explain the dietary patterns of households.

General Meal Formats for Breakfast, Lunch, and Dinner Characteristic of the Population

Breakfast[a]	Lunch[b]	Dinner[c]		
		Quick Meals	Quick to Slow Meals[d]	Slow Meals
1. Cold or cooked cereal	1. Canned/boxed meal	1. Quick meats and rolls/bread	6. Meatballs/meat sauce and pasta or other starch	8. One-pot meal: variable ingredients, sometimes with separate starch; may be boiled, stewed, or baked.
2. Home fries/french fries	2. Sandwich/hoagie	2. TV dinners	7. Various combinations of meat/fish,[e] starch(es),[f] vegetable(s)[g]	
3. Eggs and bread/cereal; home fries/french fries	3. Breakfast formats	3. Leftovers		
4. Pancakes	4. Quick-dinner formats	4. Pizza		
5. Breakfast meat and some combination of 1–4		5. Lunch formats		
6. Lunch formats				
7. Leftovers				

[a]All these meals may be eaten with or without a beverage. Beverages include coffee, tea, milk, fruit drinks, and juice. Fruit may be added to the meal.

[b]All these meals may be eaten with or without a beverage. Beverages include soda, milk, made-up powdered drinks, juice, and fruit drinks.

[c]All these meals may be eaten with or without a beverage. Beverages include iced tea, soda, made-up powdered drinks, fruit drinks, and milk. Desserts are very occasionally eaten at the time of the main meal; they are usually eaten later in the evening.

[d]Whether they are relatively quick or slow to prepare depends on whether they are made from scratch or with ready-prepared foods and on how many components they have.

[e]Beef, chicken, pork, and, less frequently, liver, turkey, and veal, among others. Usually fried; also baked/roasted in gravy, barbecued, or broiled.

[f]Potatoes, rice, macaroni variously prepared, and baked cereal products (bread, biscuits).

[g]In addition to other vegetables, such as string beans, cabbage, greens, peas, and carrots, this also includes legumes, corn, and salad, since these are all seen as vegetables or their equivalent. If cooked, usually quick boiled or stewed.

TABLE 8.2
Breakfasts Eaten by Case Study Households for One Week, in the Month Shown

Household[a]	Monday	Tuesday	Wednesday	Thursday	Friday	Saturday	Sunday
December 1977							
Mrs. Richards	Cooked cereal, Eggs	Cooked cereal	Cooked cereal	Eggs, Ham, Bread	Cooked cereal	Cooked cereal	—
Mr. Richards	Ham, Bread	Cooked cereal, Ham	Bacon		Eggs, Sausage	Ham	—
Son		Eggs and cheese, Ham	—	Sausage			—
SD	At school				Cooked cereal, Eggs, Ham	Cooked cereal	Cooked cereal
DD₁	At school		Cooked cereal, Bacon		At school	Cooked cereal, Ham	—
DD₂	Cooked cereal		Cooked cereal	Pancakes	Beefaroni (can), Bread	Cooked cereal	Cooked cereal
DD₂S	Cooked cereal	Cooked cereal	Cooked cereal		Cooked cereal	Cooked cereal	Cooked cereal
DD₃	At parents'			Pancakes	Cooked cereal	Cooked cereal	Cooked cereal
DD₃S					Eggs, Bacon	Bacon	—

200

September 1978

Jennifer

Son₁	—	At Mr. and Mrs. Richards'	Cold cereal	Cold cereal	Cold cereal	Cold cereal	Cold cereal
Son₂	At Mr. and Mrs. Richards' { Cold cereal	Cooked cereal / Eggs / Bread	Cold cereal	Cold cereal	Cold cereal	Cooked cereal / Eggs / Bread	Cold cereal
D(Gail)							
D(Gail)S							
D	At Mr. and Mrs. Richards' / Cold cereal	At Mr. and Mrs. Richards' / Bread	Eggs / Cold cereal	Cold cereal	Cold cereal	Eggs / Bread	Cold cereal

(D(Gail) / D(Gail)S: { Cold cereal)

September 1978

Rachel

Son	Cold cereal		Fruit		Cold cereal	Cold cereal	— (↑)
D					Cold cereal	Cold cereal	

September 1978

Myra

D	Pancakes	Pancakes	At aunt's	Cold cereal	Cold cereal	Cold cereal / Pancakes

July 1978

Lynne

Lynne	—	Eggs / Bread	—	Bacon / Eggs / Bread / Donuts	Sausage / Bread	—	Eggs
Eric	Beef / Eggs / Bread	—	Beef / Eggs	—	Home fries	—	Beef / Eggs / Bread
Son₁	Cold cereal / Fruit	Cold cereal	Bread	Cold cereal / Eggs	}	Cold cereal	Away
Son₂							

Note: Seasonal differences in diet and changes associated with other cycles (e.g., income cycles) are not considered here.

[a] Standard abbreviations are used for daughter (D) and son (S).

201

TABLE 8.3
Dinners Eaten by Case Study Households for One Week, During the Month Shown

Household[a]	Monday	Tuesday	Wednesday	Thursday	Friday	Saturday	Sunday
December 1977							
Mrs. Richards	Collard greens (fresh) with salt pork	Polish sausage	Fish (fresh, fried)	Lima beans (with ham and, ham hocks)	Hamburger Sauce (jar and additions)	Tuna sandwich	Chicken (fried)
Mr. Richards		Rice	Rice		Bread		Cabbage (boiled) with bacon and ham
Son	Cornbread						
SD		Peas and corn (cans)	Peas and corn (cans)	Rice		Beefaroni (can)	
DD₁							
DD₂				Rice			Rice
DD₂S						Tuna sandwich / Beefaroni	Bread
DD₃	At parents'	At parents'	At parents'	Bread		Tuna sandwich	
DD₃S	At parents'						
Only small amounts of table food eaten—aged six months →							
September 1978							
Jennifer	Stewed beef (from scratch)	Fish (fresh, fried)	Hot dogs/ sausages / Rolls	Fish sticks (fried)	Sausages	Steak (fried)	Chicken (fried)
Son₁		Macaroni (box)		Pork and beans (can)	Pork and beans (can)	Peas (can)	Peas and corn (cans)
Son₂							
D(Gail)	Rice (box)		Spaghetti and meatballs (can)	Hot dogs / Rolls / Soup	Hoagie (bought)	Rice (box)	Rice (box)
D(Gail)S		Hoagie	Sandwich		Fish sticks		
D							

202

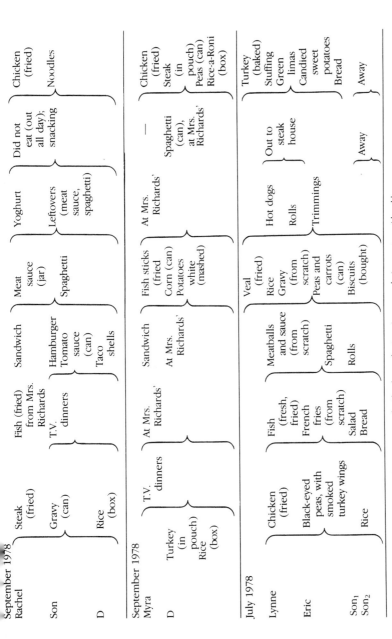

September 1978 — Rachel, Son, D

Steak (fried)	Fish (fried) from Mrs. Richards	Sandwich	Meat sauce (jar)	Yoghurt	Did not eat (out all day); snacking	Chicken (fried)
Gravy (can) / Rice (box)	T.V. dinners	Hamburger / Tomato sauce (can) / Taco shells	Spaghetti	Leftovers (meat sauce, spaghetti)	—	Noodles

September 1978 — Myra, D

T.V. dinners	At Mrs. Richards'	Sandwich	Fish sticks (fried) / Corn (can) / Potatoes white (mashed)	At Mrs. Richards'	—	Chicken (fried) / Steak (in pouch) / Peas (can) / Rice-a-Roni (box)
Turkey (in pouch) / Rice (box)		At Mrs. Richards'			Spaghetti (can), at Mrs. Richards'	

July 1978 — Lynne, Eric, Son₁, Son₂

Chicken (fried)	Fish (fresh, fried) / French fries (from scratch) / Salad / Bread	Meatballs and sauce (from scratch) / Spaghetti / Rolls	Veal (fried) / Rice / Gravy (from scratch) / Peas and carrots (can) / Biscuits (bought)	Hot dogs / Rolls / Trimmings	Out to steak house	Turkey (baked) / Stuffing / Green limas / Candied sweet potatoes / Bread
Black-eyed peas, with smoked turkey wings / Rice		Sandwich			Away	Away

Note: Seasonal differences in diet and changes associated with other cycles (e.g., income cycles) are not considered here.

ªStandard abbreviations are used for daughter (D) and son (S).

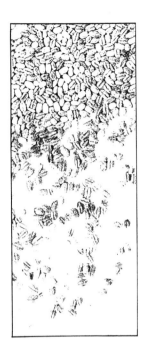

CHAPTER 9

Dietary Improvisation in an Agricultural Economy

Arjun Appadurai

With Arjun Appadurai's contribution the question of how people experience their situation, and in experiencing it act, becomes the central issue. This is a critical topic hardly considered by many researchers in nutritional anthropology, where choices, decisions, and strategies are constantly referred to but seldom explored in detail.

Rather than use more formal decision analysis, Appadurai has drawn on the writings of Schutz (1970) and Bourdieu (1977) in analyzing the complexity of the daily lives of a category of women: the different levels of their attention, and the flexibility and improvisational quality in what he has described as the intricacy, small scale, and frequency of their transactions. The richness of his presentation, however, does not lie only in his capacity through his analysis to evoke the texture and variability of the women's experience and to trace the interconnectedness of their food-related and other activities. His chapter also shows a way of incorporating equally valuable analysis of the larger-scale organization of the village (Vadi, in western India). He sets the women's activities in the context of the agricultural economy, migration and remittances, Hindu beliefs and practices, and domestic and other contingencies. He further presents a framework for analyzing the structure of diet that encompasses, among other characteristics, the importance of seasonality, and he places subsistence concerns firmly in the realm of the ongoing social life of the village, a social life that has value over and above subsistence and survival.

This chapter can be seen as one example of how all levels of experience and organization can be incorporated into a comprehensive analysis of dietary practices without fragmentation and separation of individual, household, and community. It encourages exploration of new ways to approach and analyze even apparently familiar problems in nutritional anthropology and the anthropology of food.

This chapter treats decisions concerning food in the domestic settings of an Indian village as examples of what Pierre Bourdieu has called the "regulated improvisations of the habitus" (Bourdieu 1977, 21). This means that such decisions are not best regarded either as the mechanical products of consciously held "rules" or as ad hoc and culture-free responses to raw exigency. Rather, they are culturally formed dispositions to strategize in particular ways. I will make three kinds of observation and an argument about their interconnectedness. The first concerns the relationship between the taken-for-granted aspects of decision making in a particular cultural and economic setting and those that are more in the foreground of attention (Schutz 1970). The second observation concerns the relationship between dietary decisions and other kinds of preoccupation in the daily lives of adult female household heads. The third deals with the highly permeable boundaries (both analytic and practical) between the domestic setting and the more public, large-scale factors that affect the political economy of the hearth. Though my information comes from a particular social, cultural, and historical milieu, I am quite aware that what it describes is a variant of the sort of predicament in which women find themselves in a wide variety of societies.[1]

SOME DILEMMAS OF DESCRIPTION

Self-consciousness about one's mode of presentation has recently become something of a fashion among ethnographers, following upon an earlier tendency to scrutinize the epistemological dilemmas of fieldwork. Since this chapter is written in a manner that does not fit standard modes of exposition in the study of dietary decision making, its own rhetorical stance is worth justifying.

My goal is to highlight certain qualitative, subjective, and experiential aspects of day-to-day subsistence in a particular place. I have therefore deliberately minimized the presentation of quantities, objective structures, and rules, except insofar as they illuminate the experiential side of the picture. Though I cannot provide a full justification here, my position is built on the critique of "objectivism" in

Bourdieu (1977) and of standard social science modes of measurement in Cicourel (1964) and Appadurai (1984c). I am aware that this endangers the credibility of my argument for some readers, but this seems to me preferable to dangers of the other sort.

Even if my qualitative emphasis is taken to be legitimate, it might be argued that my account is thin on actual vignettes or cases, which are often held to be the bases of descriptive ethnography. I have opted instead for a type of generalizing rhetoric, which glosses and represents cases. There is a reason for this choice as well, beyond limitations of space. Just as certain kinds of objectivist account exaggerate the significance of "rule," "structure," and "determinacy" in human action, so certain qualitative accounts, through excessive reliance on vignettes, cases, and "real" examples, create the problematic (and misleading) illusion that lived experience always has a dramatistic quality—that it is character-centered, unpredictable, and situation-based. This dramatistic illusion is, except for occasional episodes, untrue both to how most people experience their lives and to how anthropologists piece together their understandings in the field. I have therefore opted for a narrative voice that is simultaneously experiential and synoptic, and thus reflects, in a specific setting, both the typicality of experience and the experience of typicality. The ethnographic account that follows, therefore, is part of an effort to typicalize lived experience without necessarily either generalizing from, or idealizing, actual cases. Much traditional ethnography, of course, typicalizes in this way (see Marcus and Cushman 1982), but it is not so traditional to typicalize when the focus is on the qualitative side of lived experiences. In this specific regard, my effort is experimental.

One final question remains about the idiom in which I have presented this typicalizing account. Although I am concerned in some sense with the mental side of subsistence experience, I have deliberately eschewed the idioms of rational choice, of information processing, and of psychological formalisms of any sort. Instead, I have opted for a phenomenological idiom. This choice too is not simply a matter of taste. In the course of my own fieldwork, I became firmly convinced that the search for mental calculi in the heads of my informants, even if these existed, was methodologically misguided. In the face of situations of immense intricacy, fluidity, and complexity; of responses of great subtlety and speed; and of justifications that are very difficult (even for the participants) to distinguish from motives, the anthropological task of describing the sheer experience of such situations is difficult enough. The search for deeper rules, algorithms, and heuristics seems, at the least, premature. Nevertheless, I do not intend to claim that my type of account is somehow uniquely privileged or authoritative. Indeed, it is partly in the hope of raising some interesting questions for those who are committed to other modes of inquiry and to other strategies of presentation that the following account is offered.

THE VILLAGE OF VADI

Vadi is my pseudonym for the village in western India where I conducted fieldwork in 1981–82. This place is located about 25 miles southeast of the city of Pune, in the state of Maharashtra, it is about 130 miles inland (and about a four-hour train ride) from the coastal metropolis of Bombay. Vadi is a poor village by virtually any standard. It consists of about nine hundred persons who live in 193 households; approximately 30 percent are "nuclear" (*vibhakta*), while the rest are "joint" (*ekatra*) in one or another sense.[2] The total amount of cultivated land is about 880 acres, of which about 280 acres (less than 33 percent) are irrigated, largely by shared electrically powered wells (Appadurai 1984b). Mean landholdings are 4.5 acres, with mean dry landholdings being 3.1 acres and mean wet landholdings 1.4 acres.

The caste composition of Vadi is not complex. Of the 193 households, 174 belong to the Maratha caste (the dominant peasant caste of this region), while the remaining 19 households are distributed among seven other castes, including two "untouchable" castes. Vadi is the kind of village that in India and elsewhere contributes massively to urban work forces, and 104 of its households have one or more members living outside the village, either in Bombay or in Pune. The adult males among these migrants often support children and aged adults in their own urban households and thus cannot often send substantial or regular amounts of cash to their families in the village. Vadi is thus not in any simple sense a "remittance economy," though it is in a variety of ways deeply monetized.

Even the poorest of households is fundamentally tied into the cash nexus, and most households, according to widely shared local estimates, would collapse without at least a few hundred rupees a month. Apart from urban remittances, the principal sources of cash are the sale of one's own labor to others in the village and the sale of commercial crops. As for household consumption, few are self-sufficient, even in grain, and most rely on village and town shops for vegetables, spices, condiments, cooking oils, clothing, kerosene, matches, and cooking vessels. Even the wealthiest households buy some part of their grain and lentils from the market. On the other hand, there is considerable effort to strive for independence from the market in regard to food, whenever possible.

AGRICULTURAL LIVELIHOOD

But for a few virtually destitute men and women, who depend entirely on the goodwill of others for their subsistence, all the households in Vadi rely either wholly or in part on agriculture in order to subsist. Agriculture in this part of the Deccan plateau is both a low-technology and a high-risk enterprise. Apart from the approximately fifty-seven wells that are powered by small electric or diesel motors, the technology of agriculture relies on animal traction, human labor, and wooden and steel tools that have probably changed in the last few centuries, but only in matters of detail. Modern fertilizers and pesticides are increasingly used for commercial crops, particularly vegetables. Rainfall in Vadi is probably less than twenty-five inches in most years and is sharply seasonal. The peak period of rainfall in normal years is during June, July, August, and September, which accounts for about 75 percent of the total. October and November usually account for about 15 percent, the months from December to March for about 3 percent, and April and May for about 7 percent.

The principal subsistence crops are sorghum (*jvari*) and millet (*bajri*), and most villagers grow at least some of each. In addition, there is a large inventory of other cultigens. Small amounts of wheat and rice are grown. The principal commercial crops are onions, green peas, sugarcane, and fresh coriander. Also important, but more for consumption than for sale, are a variety of lentils and pulses, many kinds of greens, a few fruits, some oilseeds, and such vegetables as tomatoes, green chilies, garlic, and carrots. Finally, a few farmers devote small parts of their plots to animal fodder. All the crops grown principally for sale, as well as all the vegetables, require irrigated land.

There are two major cropping seasons: the *kharif* season, from June to October (which relies on the monsoon rains), when both sorghum and millet are grown; and the *rabi* (winter) season, which runs from November to January, when the bulk of the irrigation-dependent, market-oriented farming is done. The hot season, which runs from March to May, is the most taxing, because wells run dry, harvests of grain and vegetables have been depleted either through consumption or sale, and expenses for rituals (especially marriages) tend to peak. It is during this hot season that the ritual and the production years reach their highest (followed by their lowest) points of intensity. In May, the ritual cycle subsides, the land is prepared for the following year, and the yearning for the June rains deepens.

WOMEN AND THE PROVISION OF FOOD

Food is a subject of special salience in the Hindu world. Since this chapter focuses on the improvisational aspects of domestic subsistence, I shall say something about food as a culturally organized domain of significance in Hindu India. Much of great value has been written on this topic (Khare 1976a, 1976b; Marriott 1968, 1976; Stone 1978), and there is surely no need for yet another demonstration that food is part of specialized moral and medical taxonomies; that it ties together ideas of impurity, exchange, and rank; that the logic of the hearth is the logic of the Hindu cosmos in miniature; or that there is a symbolic dimension to food production and processing. Much of this is true for Vadi, though only some of the ways in which these cultural assumptions take shape in the village are addressed in this chapter. In my own previous work, I have sought to contextualize these kinds of significance in problems of micropolitics (Appadurai 1981), of large-scale cultural change (Appadurai 1984c), and of the political economy of entitlement (Appadurai 1984a) in India. What we do need are better accounts of the ways in which these significances are parts of lived local experience, of specific forms of sociality, and of regular improvisatory practice. It is to the latter need that this chapter is addressed.

Throughout my discussion, the problem of domestic food provision is viewed from the female perspective. But a word of clarification is in order. The women of Vadi are neither economically nor existentially in identical situations. Some rely more than others on selling their own agricultural labor. Some have husbands and sons with them, while others head their village households because their husbands are away in Bombay or Pune. Some are actively involved in farming on their plots, while others, either because they are landless or because they come from larger or wealthier households, do not labor in the fields. Some work under the eye of older women (mothers and mothers-in-law), while others are on their own. Finally, some are too young to bear household responsibilities, while others, because they are poor, infirm, or indifferent, play no role in household decisions. These are important differences, and a full examination would take them carefully into account. But many women are involved in the management of households, rely on produce from their fields as well as on income from the sale of cash crops and their own labor, and are perpetually in one or another form of debt. These are the women—ranging in age from twenty to sixty, all from the dominant Maratha caste, and whose households do not have more than five acres of land— whose voices inform this chapter. Even among them there are important differences, such as the presence or absence of their husbands, the number and health of their children, the age and demands of their parents or in-laws, the prospects for marriage of their sons and daughters, and their own physical strength and health in relation to agricultural labor. Yet, these women have enough in common for my purposes. The resources on which they draw, the problems they face, the language and style of their narratives of their lives, the approach they take to juggling the claims upon them, are similar enough to justify the lumping that must inevitably occur in such an analysis as this one.[3]

Providing food for the daily needs of the household is a responsibility that falls on the shoulders of women in Vadi, but it is a task that is not defined by rigid conceptions or measures of "need" or "requirement." Rather, it is framed by the interaction between a variety of seasonalities and periodicities as they are perceived and engaged in by particular female food providers. Some of these periodicities represent collective, large-scale, and socially set rhythms, such as the cycle of the seasons; the life cycle of specific cultigens; the ups and downs of the labor market; the vagaries of price in the vegetable markets of Saswad (the small market and administrative town about three miles from Vadi), Pune, and Bombay; and the rhythm of regional, village, and lineage festivals and rituals. Other periodicities are centripetal and involve trajectories that are idiosyncratic and variable from household to household—marriages and deaths, with their attendant high expenses for ritual; medical emergencies, small and large; cash flows from urban wages, vegetable sales, or sales of labor, which vary not just because of market factors but also in relation to individual energies and choices; biographical periodicities that affect the medical, ritual, and educational needs of children, adult dependents, and adult workers in the household; the complex periodicities of debts, small and large, to banks, vegetable wholesalers, potential affines, neighbors, and kinsmen; and so forth.

In the context of all these periodicities and seasonalities, the struggle to feed members of the household adequately involves the continuous effort to improvise acceptable allocations of time, energy, and money against contextually defined ideas of maternal concern, social standing, and moral propriety. It is the experiential texture of this continuous effort that I wish to capture, at least in part, in the rest of this chapter.

The provision of food in this context entails the juggling of available items (itself a function of the agricultural seasons and of

the availability of cash for purchases when necessary) against routine and not-so-routine demands, within the framework of a basic
stock of knowledge about food purchasing, processing, cooking,
and eating. This knowledge is widely shared as regards recipes;
rituals; the needs of the sick, the pregnant, the aged; the shifting
prices of foodstuffs; and so on. It is necessarily less shared or standardized in regard to such centripetal and individual factors as individual tastes and income flows. Indeed, it might even be appropriate to call this latter sort of knowledge "information" and reserve
the term "knowledge" for the former, shared elements.[4]

THE STRUCTURE OF THE DIET

Against this backdrop, the structure of the diet may be described as
modular, stratified, and *seasonal*. Let me explain these terms and
use them to provide the material context for the strategies of
domestic food provision. The building blocks of daily meals are
millet- or sorghum-based pan-roasted bread (*bhakri*), an item so
basic that its name provides the colloquial term for food; seasonally
available vegetables, principally eggplant, onions, garlic, and a variety of greens; soups made of either farm-grown or store-bought
lentils of several sorts, principally yellow split peas (*harbara*); sea-
sonings that are themselves used in various standard combinations
(these include fresh ingredients, such as coconut, coriander, garlic,
red or green chilies, and mustard seed, with vegetable oils as their
base); chick-pea flour, which has almost the status of a staple; and
various hot preserves (*chatni*) made principally of garlic and red
chilies. These constitute the modular basis of meals.

Playing a less important role, because they are used either in
very small quantities or too occasionally, are meat (usually mutton);
fish; chicken; eggs (from household hens); milk (usually from domestic goats, but also from cows and buffaloes); and a variety of
sweet, festive preparations whose base is rice, sugar, milk, wheat,
chick-pea flour, and shortening or clarified butter in various combinations that are both labor and money intensive. Also in a category
of their own are tea and sugar, the constant accompaniments of any

kind of social activity (sometimes used with milk). Finally, some men (and a few women) smoke *bidis* (native cigarettes), and many women chew a mild narcotic called *mishri*, which is held to be a stimulant and an appetite depressant. These latter items are comestibles but hardly foods. Children, whenever possible, purchase biscuits, toffee, candies, and savories from the two village stores, as do adults less frequently. Children and adults get small quantities of some fruit (mangoes, figs, oranges, bananas), subject to heavy seasonal and wealth variations.

These sets of foods may be described as modular because they represent a group of elements that can be combined into daily, weekly, monthly, and seasonal patterns that are either complex (and therefore both satisfying and nutritious, as far as I can judge) or exceedingly spare and simple. The elementary meal is a few pieces of sorghum or millet bread (*bhakri*) with an extremely hot, concentrated, but cheaply produced *chatni*, usually made of just garlic and red chilies with salt and water. The term used for food, especially by men and women living very close to the bone, is *bhakar-chatni*, referring to just this combination. Other elements can be added progressively to make meals of increasing richness and range. Thus a decent midday meal, especially for working men and women, would include several large pieces of bread, a lentil soup (*amti* or *varan*), a pan-fried vegetable, and some spicy pickle or condiment. The vegetable and soup items can be made with more or less elaborate spice combinations, and they can be heavy on water and cheap spices or on oil and expensive ones. In the fields, however, most meals consist of just bread and one substantial accompaniment. The most important component of certain routine snack foods is tapioca (*sabudana*), which is also used on "fast" days. Peanuts play a central role in many vegetable or lentil preparations, and I suspect they are the most reliable sources of protein in the diet in Vadi.

The inventory of foods is also stratified insofar as there is an ordering of the modules, which is fairly explicit. The millet breads form the base (regular, plain, low-cost), along with the chick-pea-flour-based preparation and *chatnis*. The vegetable and lentil preparations constitute the second tier (with an internal subhierarchy based on the complexity of spices used in them). The top tier is based on animal protein and such high-fat and high-calorie items as meat, sweets, milk products, and eggs. This part of the hierarchy is based on what are regarded as appropriate foods for important ritual events, such as marriages, funerals, and offerings to deities. (More shall be said about feasting in another part of this chapter.) The point about stratification is that it links the modules both to seasonal variation and to stratification in the social sense, since the wealthier households more frequently have combinations of modules involving higher-ranked foodstuffs and preparations.

Seasonality is the most obvious part of this dietary structure. The basic grains are harvested at different times: millet mainly in the *kharif* season, sorghum in both the *kharif* and *rabi* seasons, wheat only in the winter season, and rice at the end of the wet season. The end of the winter and the beginning of the hot season is when the range of vegetables is greatest, because of the irrigation factor, which determines when onions, peas, eggplant, and chilies may be harvested. Lentils and peanuts, because of their preservability, are available on the market throughout the year, as are the basic food grains, spices, oils, flours, salt, and sugar. But for those whose cash income is small and unpredictable, and whose own holdings are tiny and unproductive, foods on the market are not always within their grasp to even out the seasonalities of their own production and the gaps between the harvests of basic grains, as well as between those of vegetables and lentils. These gaps, which occur often at times of greatest need, are closed by contracting short- or long-term debts.

The modular, stratified, and seasonal aspects of the dietary process are deeply interconnected in the experience of the women who are responsible for domestic subsistence in Vadi. The combination of modules into low- and high-quality meals is not only a function of the rank of the modules that are used but also of the seasonalities bearing on the household in question. Festive meals require high-ranking foods and complex modular combinations insofar as the household in question is able to produce them under seasonal constraints. Even ordinary daily meals, whether served at home or in the fields, can be based on very elementary modules or can be complex combinations, depending on the seasonal state of the household in question. There is no set number of meals in the day for a given household. Frequency varies across households (depending on who works and at what distance from home, as well as on the many other factors already mentioned) and within households, where there is a definite tendency to provide multiple, complex, high-ranking food combinations (as far as possible) to workers over nonworkers, to men over women, and to children over nonworking adults. As far as I can see, these latter three criteria are ranked as I have listed them, though a variety of contingencies (such as illness, domestic violence, or the appearance of important guests) may change their ordering.

Let us now move back from the components of the dietary structure to the larger context of women's lives. Women in Vadi stand at the interphase between the production and the consumption processes as far as food is concerned. They are actively involved in a large range of agricultural tasks, either in their own fields or, for cash wages, in the fields of others. These tasks include weeding a variety of crops, which is spread through the rainy and winter seasons; planting most of the vegetable crops; harvesting the grain crops and the vegetable crops; and threshing, winnowing, husking, drying, and storing all the cultigens. In addition, they are responsible for the care of the smaller domestic animals (goats and chickens). They do some of the local selling of vegetable and grain surpluses and much of the shopping at the village store. Women whose husbands are away are responsible for monitoring any sharecropping arrangement that they might have for their own plots, which often includes giving their own labor at key times. Finally, and not least, they must get water for domestic use from wells or streams, wash clothes and utensils, collect firewood or manure for fuel, and tend all dependent children. Somewhere in the midst of all these tasks, most of which have irregular and uncertain periodicities, they must think about feeding the members of their households. The experiential quality of this dietary dimension of their daily responsibilities can best be discussed under two headings, which occupy the following two sections of this chapter. These sections also refine, qualify, and contextualize some of the observations made so far.

SCALE, INTRICACY, AND FREQUENCY IN WOMEN'S TRANSACTIONS

One implication of the kind of situation that has been sketched thus far is that the nature of tasks, decisions, and transactions in which women in Vadi are engaged is distinctive. This characteristic quality, which has to do with the special *scale, intricacy*, and *frequency* of their interactions, is what most distinguishes their situation from that of adult men in comparable households. These are distinct but interrelated qualities, and I deal with them sequentially, starting with scale.

Although there are few areas of subsistence in which women do not have some role, they are typically involved in smaller-scale issues than their husbands, fathers, and sons. This can be seen in a variety of dimensions. Take the matter of money. Typically, women do not handle large sums, either because the money is doled out in small (often unpredictable) amounts by their wage-earning husbands or sons or because they themselves are rarely involved in larger-scale payments for their own labor, usually being paid by the day for most of the work they do. This is true for their agricultural labor (such as weeding, planting, or threshing) and for the domestic chores they sometimes do for other women in the village, such as plastering house walls with manure, husking grain, sorting onions, and picking stones out of lentils. Finally, when they are involved directly in selling commercial crops, it is usually in the sale of small amounts of vegetables, left over from household consumption, on a seasonal basis at the nearby market in Saswad. In all these cases, the amounts of money that pass through female hands rarely exceed 100 rupees at a time. (In 1981–82 the U.S. $ fluctuated between 9 and 10 rupees on the foreign exchange market.) This upper ceiling is set by average remittances from working husbands in cities. The lower limit, which represents the far more frequently handled sums, is in the range of the 4 to 8 rupees a day that women make for agricultural labor, depending on the season and the task. In between these parameters are the proceeds of low-level local sale of vegetables. Not only do women deal with small sums of money gained and spent in a series of small dealings (to be described below), they are, by extension, involved in allocative moves over smaller periods, though they are frequently aware of issues that span weeks, months, even years. That is, women may, and do, have in the back of their minds problems of grain shortages, sharecropping contracts, forthcoming marriages, and ritual commitments that may place the horizons of their attention over an extended temporal landscape. But the bulk of their energy is necessarily devoted to matters that recur in a shorter time frame. This is nowhere truer than in the domain of food, which I shall come to shortly.

Further, the social universe in which women are embedded on a daily basis is on the whole restricted to a small number of persons and to a space that is closely tied to their houses and neighborhoods, by comparison to the numerical and spatial scope of the social worlds of adult men. This is not, of course, to deny that women often deal with strangers, that they often go long distances to work in someone else's fields or their own, that they sometimes maintain links with kinsmen and affines in villages far away, or that they occasionally conduct religiously inspired journeys to places outside the district. All this is true, yet, when compared with men (as we shall see in the next section on the sociality of subsistence), women's dealings take place in a numerically and spatially more confined world.

Closely linked to the small scale of the interactional world of women is its intricacy.[5] This is a somewhat subtler point that is closer to the central thrust of this chapter. Women deal not only with fewer people, over smaller units of time, with smaller amounts of cash or kind, but their dealings are more intricate when compared with those of men. That is, over any given short period, such as a few hours, a day, or even a week, women are likely to be shifting their attention very rapidly, and they are likely to be engaged in attending to several tasks at once. This means that their attention has to be more intricately and more involutedly allocated between foreground and background issues.

This intricacy is not only a function of the small scale and high turnover of many of the things they are handling but also arises because the handling of these various tasks is not spatially segregated, as it often is with men's work. Thus, women at market are often minding children at the same time; when they go out to gather firewood, they might need to attend to their goats (and possibly their children) simultaneously. Sometimes all these tasks are constrained by the objective of getting food to husbands or sons in the fields. Frequently, such a heavily overlaid and intricate schedule is further complicated by critical tasks (such as being at someone else's house or fields for work) that cannot easily be manipulated. Intricacy has another, more literal dimension as well. Women are frequently involved in mending clothes, fixing small tools, making minor repairs to the house, tending chronic ailments of animals, constructing temporary ritual designs of chalk inside or outside the home, and other activities that require focusing intensely on micro-designs, whether physical, aesthetic, or structural. Examples of the intricacy of women's dealings can be multiplied, and more will be said about this quality in relation to food at the end of this section and in relation to sociality in the next.

The frequency of women's engagements adds the final twist to the picture of small-scale, intricate actions. They must shift from locus to locus (from field to house to stream to market to temple to someone else's threshing ground); from transaction to transaction (from the village shop to the doctor to a sharecropping partner to a sick friend); from social frame to social frame (from dyadic nurture of an infant to friendly rebuke of a daughter to an ongoing quarrel with a neighbor to an ambiguous relationship with a friend to a humiliating encounter with a creditor to an abusive relationship with an employer); and from medium to medium (from dealings in food to dealings in cash to dealings in pots and pans to dealings in animal manure). Such shifts, and many others like them, mean that the transactional world of women in Vadi is not only composed of small-scale dealings, of intricate and interweaving demands for attention and action, but also that the small scale and intricacy of transactions are compounded by the high frequency of shifts, in the venue, frame, and medium, of these transactions. Together, these changes add up to a world that is, in regard to the conscious attention of women, miniaturized, fluid, and fast moving.

Let us now use one extended example to look more closely at the implications of these qualities for the domestic handling of foods. It is based on my interaction on a day in April 1982 with a woman called S., who lives with her husband in Vadi. She is somewhat better off than many women in the village. She and her husband still control their small plots of land and are therefore able to assert authority over both their sons (one is unmarried and lives with them, while the other lives nearby with his wife).

"I am very weary today," S. begins. "Therefore I did not cook at all. In a little while I am going to make a little spiced rice [*fodnichi bhat*]." She then says she is going to get some cooked vegetable (*bhaji*) from her daughter-in-law, who lives nearby. Coming back with some lentil soup and sorghum bread, she continues: "Yesterday was an important ritual day, and someone from every house had to make the journey to Shikhat Singhnapur [a nearby pilgrimage site]. They all had to be given *bhaji puri* [a bread and vegetable combination] and *puran poli* [a special sweet bread] for this journey."

At this juncture her husband shows up and says he is off to the pilgrimage site. He asks S. whether she has any *bhakri* (bread, here loosely meaning "food"); she says she does not but will go and see if someone else has any. Meanwhile, her husband goes off to try to collect some money owed to him by another man.

S. then states that she has only one small plot (*vavar*), from which she just got a harvest of onions and sold it for Rs. 900. She intends, she says, to dole this money out to her sons. She gave Rs. 250 to one of them yesterday, who, instead of buying grain, bought a cot. She was so furious that he went back and got one bag of grain. "Now the remaining money has to be given to people in Saswad [the nearby market town]. I had to leave my nose-ring with a doctor who is giving me injections and pills for my health, and I have to give him some money and reclaim it."

Her husband then returns with Rs. 10. S. gets angry with him and asks how he dare come back with this paltry sum. She takes out a Rs. 100 note, and he gives her Rs. 70 back. She then gives him two pieces of bread for his trip.

This vignette is unusual in some respects, for S. clearly has more authority in her household than many women in Vadi do, though they are not generally reticent about expressing their views. Also, the relatively large sums of money that are being handled here reflect the fact that harvests of commercial vegetables occur in April. But so do the demands of debtors, of ritual, and of less than provident males like S.'s son, who indulges his desire for a Western-style cot over a stock of grain. But most of all, this episode illustrates the small flows of food between households that are going on all the time in Vadi and the very complex transactional frames within which they occur. Finally, this vignette illustrates very nicely the intercalibration of ritual, market, and debt periodicities that frames dietary decisions at the household level. Also, though S. is different from many women in not having small children to feed, she does illustrate the flexibility of daily food production in the house and the weariness (*kantala*) that sometimes pushes women to simplify their own cooking and draw on kin and neighbors for short-term food needs. The social prerequisites of such flexibility are dealt with in the next section. Finally, for reasons that were not entirely clear to me, S. told her husband that she had no food to give him, though she had just gotten some from her daughter-in-law, part of which she did subsequently give him. This was clearly a small move in some ongoing micropolitical dealings in food in this extended family (Appadurai 1981).

Small-scale food flows are not only to be seen in the amicable borrowing of cooked food. (The term for such borrowing is *usne*, which means any friendly loan that does not entail interest: It can involve food, money, tools, or virtually anything else.) It also goes on between households in the matter of vegetables, grain, tea, sugar, and milk. But small-scale food transactions are mainly seen in the village grocery shops, where women come in all the time to buy oil, grain, lentils, spices, tea, or sugar in amounts (often a handful) that seem unbelievably small to the outsider's eye and that are doubtless economically inefficient purchases. But given the small-denomination, high-velocity circulation of money through female hands, there is frequently no alternative to such transactions.

At the same time, women are continuously monitoring (though here it is very difficult to generalize about the degree of conscious attention with which they do this) the quantity and nature of what is coming off their own plots, the market prices and availabilities of what is not in their own harvests, and the current or prospective arrival of visitors and guests, especially in the postharvest festival season. In doing this, they rely on their experience from past years about how long their basic grain stocks might last (the critical question) and how long stocks of other staples (if such stocks exist) can be expected to last. Finally, in making daily dietary decisions, the flow of money from any sort of income, as well as the degree of pressure to pay off what seem to be never-ending debts, has to be constantly assessed, as do the choices of what to cook, how to cook it, how much to cook, and when to cook it.

It is in the context of this sort of small-scale, fluid, and microscopic manipulation of food flows and claims that women are constantly adjusting the modular, stratified, and seasonal structure of the dietary inventory that I discussed in the preceding section. At all times, the pressures of sociality (whatever they may be) have to be weighed against the contingencies of the domestic economy itself. In this conjuncture, all women have a clear idea of what they might like to cook from meal to meal, from day to day, and from season to season. But what they actually cook is the continuously shifting (and indirect) product of the interweaving of other pressures through the hearth. Both the sources of, and the solutions to, some of these dilemmas lie outside the household in transdomestic forms of sociality, and it is to the discussion of these forms that I now turn.

THE SOCIALITY OF SUBSISTENCE

Studies of domestic dietary decisions too often convey the impression that domestic food decisions occur in functional and psychological isolation from the larger world of production and community life. From the vantage point of women in Vadi, a variety of social processes penetrates the hearth constantly. But equally, the requirements of food provision press men and women into particular ways of being social.

I have already mentioned that small-scale loans of food are an important aspect of life in Vadi. These movements of food between households are part of a very complex world of social relations, principally between women. In the first place, they reflect the widespread recognition by women that without such small flows (reciprocal at least in theory and over the long run) most households would find themselves occasionally in distress. For the kinds of periodicities and contingencies discussed throughout this chapter imply that there will frequently be needs for such loans.

But the fact is that such needs themselves arise because of the larger social worlds within which the households of Vadi are embedded. When the out-migrant man or men of the household come to visit Vadi, both the pace of social life and commensal complexity increase. Other men are likely to visit, and the resident male will probably extend invitations to them to stay and have a meal, frequently without any advance notice. Such contingencies can be fairly common for those women whose husbands work in Pune (which is only about twenty-five miles away), as frequent as once every week or two. In the case of men who work in Bombay, the visits are likely to be lengthier but less frequent, and they usually coincide with peak periods of agricultural or ritual activity, most often in April, May, and June. Sometimes, these periods coincide with increases in cash flow, since the absent men like to show their largess when they visit, however incapable they are of sending regular remittances during the rest of the year. At the very least, such unexpected entertainment of guests means that tea (with milk and sugar if at all possible) must be offered.

It is in these circumstances that, if a household has run out of its own sugar, someone (usually a young son or daughter) must run to the store for a small-scale transaction. If the woman of the house does not have her own goat, she needs to have one or more relationships with women who do so that she can get small amounts of milk at short notice. Such small-scale transactions in milk, sugar, and sometimes tea leaves are the most frequent and humble of these interhousehold movements of food. Maintaining good relations with friends, kinsmen, or affines, especially in one's immediate neighborhood, is critical if one is to have access to these forms of credit. One way to assure such access is, of course, to be responsive to such needs on the part of others whenever possible. This form of pressure to maintain social relations in one's neighborhood is, of course, magnified when one wishes to borrow more substantial items, such as grain, vegetables, oil, or lentils.

Another avenue through which the larger world of Vadi is articulated with household dietary flows and contingencies is the ritual process. Vadi is a thoroughly Hindu village, and its Hinduism is deeply embedded in the geography and religious history of Maharashtra, particularly in the songs of the poet–saints of the medieval period and the shrines of the regional incarnations of the great gods of Hinduism. Village families make pilgrimages to a variety of sacred places, some of which (like Alandi, Jejuri, and Pandharpur) are more cosmopolitan in their reach and of others which are more narrow in their significance, such as the temples of Kalubai and Khandoba. In the course of the year, there are smaller, village-based observances dedicated to a variety of deities, some calendric and some timed by individual households. In addition, there are important days during which ancestor shrines (*pitr*) in the fields are given food offerings or lineage deities in the village are worshipped. There are six shrines in the village, but the one at which the most important collective celebrations (including the major village festival of the year, simply referred to as *urus*) take place is the Vitthala temple.

In addition to these celebrations, which are inspired by the particular stories and theories associated with specific deities, there are a large variety of life-cycle rituals, the most important of which are the massive feasts associated with birth and death. The common element in these ritual events—whether they are collective or domestic, calendric or life-cycle, large-scale or small-scale, oriented to fertility or to prosperity—is the place of special foods in them. The gods and the ancestors, depending upon the context, demand special foods, the most important of which is *puran poli* (a whole-wheat pan-fried bread with a jaggery and clarified butter filling), the quintessential festive food. At such large-scale social events as marriage and death ceremonies, the meals tend to be maximal elaborations of normal domestic fare. Especially at the height of the marriage and festival season, but to some extent throughout the year, women are frequently engaged in preparing one or another kind of festive food, either for themselves and their immediate coresidents, as contributions for collective offerings to various deities, or for taking along for subsistence and for offering on pilgrimages. Marriages (which cluster together after the winter harvest in the hot months of April and May) and deaths occasion large-scale feasts (involving from a hundred to a thousand guests). At such times, the domestic economies of the host household (and, to some extent, the host lineage) are completely subordinated to the exigencies of public commensality. Such events leave their mark, through mechanisms of financial and social debt, during the months and even the years to come.

The point of the relationship between this complex and differentiated ritual process and the domestic dietary process is that it is multidimensional. It involves an ongoing set of demands for special, high-cost, labor-intensive foods, and sometimes for large amounts of them. But these demands cut both ways. On the one hand, they represent an additional source of stress for women who are already dealing with a large number of exigencies. On the other hand, they represent a deeply meaningful form of give and take, that provides, in the Hindu world, the stuff of social relations at levels ranging from the family to the village and beyond. In addition, insofar as these special foods are directed to deities, ancestors, and spirits who dwell in houses, in village temples, in fields, in wells, in streams, and in larger regional shrines, they are part of the great Hindu cycle of dealings with divinity, whose reward is the productivity of the land, the fertility of women, and the prosperity of the household.

In thus responding to the exigencies of the ritual calendar, women in particular are simultaneously interacting on three levels with the world around them: with the world as a source of demands and limits, both logistical and social; with the world as a place of persons (deities, kinsmen, friends, guests, and even strangers), who require special treatment but who are one's own source of security in ways that are direct and indirect, short- and long-term, specific and diffuse; and, finally, with the world as a scheme of divine persons and forces that return, transvalued, the sustenance given to them, both as *prasad* (sacred food) and as prosperity. From the practical point of view, ritual and festive food, its preparation, its exchange, and its consumption, constitutes the moral center of the habitus of the villagers of Vadi. For it is in the context of ritual food that the harsh reality of economizing (*kat-kasar karne*) in an agricultural milieu is repeatedly transformed into the experience of meaningful sociality and moral renewal. This sort of ritual-inspired food preparation best captures the double edge of all women's work in a peasant society such as Vadi: toilsome and distracting on the one hand, but pivotal to the reproduction of the group as a moral entity on the other.

Women recognize this complex relationship of food to social and moral renewal in the inverse of feasting, fasting (*upavas*). Fasting is a very important aspect of practical religion in Hindu India, and so it is in Vadi. Most households have at least one member who fasts at least one day a week, and if it is just one person who fasts it is likely to be the senior woman. However, men and boys also fast, usually in association with their voluntary devotion to a specific deity. For adult women, such regularized fasting is also usually connected to a vow (*navas*) to some particular (usually regional) deity related to some specific boon, either granted or prayed for. Fasting involves, as elsewhere in India, renouncing grains—not all food—and relying on other foods. In Vadi, as elsewhere in Maharashtra, the standard "fasting food" is tapioca (*sabudana*) made into a sort of stew (*khichdi*), sometimes supplemented by fruit. Even fasting can be an occasion for sociality, since friends or kinswomen sometimes bring each other these foods on fast ending days. Thus even the fasting periodicities of women who live or work in proximity can affect each other significantly.

Finally, the small- and large-scale provision of food to households other than one's own, sometimes in small and spontaneous ways and at other times in predictable and more substantial forms, is tied to subsistence through another kind of sociality, the informal female work group. The term for such work groups (whether of men or of women) is *varangula*. When men use this word it refers to a precisely structured, enduring agreement involving at least two and usually no more than four men, to pool bullocks and tools for specific agricultural activities, mainly involving the beginning of the farming year. Women's *varangula* groups, however, are larger because the tasks in which they are involved (like onion planting or harvesting) demand more workers. They are also more variable and fluid in their composition and are more closely tied to friendships and kinship relationships that are fortified by spatial proximity. Information about the need for such work groups, the likelihood of being asked to participate in them, and the ability to draw on smaller, informal versions of them to do minor household tasks depends on keeping these networks lubricated through the reciprocities of food.

Friendships in this female world are very complex, conflicted, and pivotal. For women must maintain relations with other women (whether kinswomen or neighbors) who constitute their more or less permanent local support groups; the monitors of their own domestic lives; the potential sources of nasty gossip, but also of critical support when it is needed; and the keys to vital information and opportunities for participation in remunerative work groups. Maintaining these networks, often in the face of other pressing demands on one's resources, is the other modality through which production and consumption are socially interdigitated. For one's friendships with one's female neighbors, like the demands of gods, guests, and husbands, entail expenditures of time and energy that women experience as exhausting. Yet, as sources of compassion, loans, moral support at critical moments, protection from irate husbands, information about work, and just as shoulders to cry on, these friendships are the mainstay of adult female life in Vadi. But keeping up these friendships also requires a willingness to make small loans of food, to share food freely when one is in the fields with a work group, and to give a share of cooked food to lineage, neighborhood, or village festivities.

In all these ways, the dietary decisions of the hearth are deeply connected to the worlds of the neighborhood, the fields, the marketplace, and even to the religious life of the region. Each of these other arenas implies a different form and kind of sociality, and each one is Janus faced, representing harsh budgetary exigencies on one side and moral security and social standing on the other. This is the dual link between sociality and subsistence in the lived experience of the women of Vadi.

CONCLUSION: EXIGENCY AND IMPROVISATION IN DIETARY STRATEGY

I have sought to capture the texture of domestic dietary strategies, as I construe it, in the lives of some women in Vadi. Two analytic points have been made in the course of this descriptive account. The first is that women's transactions are small-scale, intricate, and frequent. The second is that if we trace the paths of women's attention we are inevitably forced to see that dietary decisions are intimately connected to problems that have to do with other larger and more public arenas of social life. It remains now to ask what the implications of these two points are for an adequate characterization of the quality of dietary strategies at the domestic level.

Schutz (1970) whom I cite in the first paragraph of this chapter, makes a distinction, in his account of how human beings render some parts of their environment more relevant than others, between "theme" and "horizon" (Schutz 1970). The former is an element that is in the foreground of the attention of the actor and is subject to conscious scrutiny and manipulation. The horizon consists of whatever sets the backdrop, the frame, the boundaries of the actor's ongoing (and ever-shifting) mental landscape. Looked at from this perspective, the first conclusion to be drawn from my description is that dietary decisions are rarely explicit, systematic, conscious, or set apart from other issues in the way that many analyses imply. Using Schutz's terms, and following the description I have constructed, it should be noted that the relationship between "horizon" and "theme," between background and foreground issues, is continuously shifting for the women of Vadi. On the whole, and except when there is a truly unusual configuration of circumstances, daily dietary choice is made in what Gladwin and Murtaugh (1980) would call a "pre-attentive manner," and dietary issues remain in the background of women's attention. In this regard, dietary decisions are no more privileged than the other activities in which women must engage, and they move into the foreground of women's attention only insofar as, and for so long as, they present a more pressing or more puzzling choice than some other one.

This is not a peculiar artifact of mental structure in Vadi. It is a function of the sorts of issues, far transcending the hearth and the meal, in which dietary strategies are embedded. At the same time, women can carry on the task of providing food to the members of their household in a largely pre-attentive manner because an important part of their habitus is a mental inventory, a stance, and a disposition that allow them to deploy their shifting assets effectively. Such strategizing is neither a mechanical following of "rules" nor an ad hoc and culture-free response to exigency. It is an example of what Bourdieu has called "regulated improvisation," a characteristic of important aspects of social life in many stable societies. But it seems especially true of peasant societies, more still of their domestic settings, and is nowhere better exemplified than in the daily strategies of women for feeding their families.

NOTES

Acknowledgments: This chapter was written while the author was a Fellow at the Center for Advanced Study in the Behavioral Sciences, Stanford, California. Financial support during this period was provided by the National Science Foundation (BNS 8011494) and by the University of Pennsylvania. Fieldwork in Maharashtra, India, during 1981 and 1982 was supported by the National Science Foundation, the American Institute for Indian Studies, and the Social Science Research Council. Carol Breckenridge provided useful comments and criticisms on an earlier draft of this chapter, as did the editors.

1. The argument of this chapter will be elaborated and contextualized in a forthcoming collection of essays by the author, tentatively titled *Improvisation and Experience in an Agricultural Society*. Since there are very few citations in the text of this chapter, I should note that I have been influenced, in a variety of ways, by the following scholars and studies. On the status of working women in India, I have learned a great deal from Gulati (1981), Miller (1981), Papanek (1979, 1984) and Sharma (1980). N. S. Jodha's numerous microlevel analyses of agriculture in semiarid environments in India have provided suggestive descriptions and hypotheses. Chambers, Longhurst, and Pacey (1981) made me aware of the complexities of seasonality. Finally, my approach to human action, social forms, and lived experience owes a great deal to Bourdieu (especially Bourdieu 1977) and to Schutz (particularly Schutz 1970).

2. Rural speakers of Marathi have a clear lexical way to distinguish "household" (*ghar*) from "family" (*kutumb*). The term *ghar* is, pragmatically speaking, used to refer to the physical dwelling (house); the group of people living together in it; and to domestic aspects of life as opposed to public ones, as in *ghar-kam* (house-work). *Kutumb* is, by contrast, a technical term that is not often used except in formal interview situations, normally to refer to an agnatically related and coresident group of kinsmen with a living male head. But when livelihood is a shared concern among a group of persons, however complex or indirect their kinship links, the term *ghar* (household) is likely to be used. When referring to co-members of a household, who live in separate houses (as when men are away in Bombay), *ghar* may or may not be used, depending on whether the pragmatic emphasis is on physical dwellings or on budgetary units. Finally, the terms *ekatra* (united) or *vibhakta* (separate) refer to the commensal and productive relations of agnates, not to physical dwellings: Thus, a household with loci in Bombay and Vadi may nevertheless be a "joint" family (*ekatra kutumb*).

3. The data for this chapter come from informal observations and conversations, as well as taped interviews, with women in about twenty households in Vadi. I owe a special debt to Mrs. S. Gogate, my assistant, whose rapport with some of these women helped me to grasp things I would never have understood otherwise. But it is to the women themselves, who improvise domestic security in extremely trying circumstances, that this chapter is dedicated.

4. In distinguishing "knowledge" from "information," I wish to contrast two ways in which actors apprehend their environments. While knowledge

has to do with retrospect, with regularity, with structure, with generalizations, and with the taken for granted, information involves prospect, irregularity, events, particulars, and conscious attention. From the point of view of cultural and social sharing, knowledge is what one has (or thinks one has), whereas information is what one seeks. A full anthropological account of these two categories would be very complex and would, among other things, note that it is within particular frameworks of knowledge that the nature of information itself is defined.

5. The use of the term "intricacy" here is intended to characterize the experiential aspect or aspects of women's work in many societies, whose behavioral complexity has frequently been noted. It also overlaps to some degree with the use of the terms "intricacy" and "complexity" in Douglas and Gross (1981) and in Douglas (1984). However, Douglas's emphasis is on the macrointricacy of rule systems, whereas my emphasis is on the microintricacy of attention and action, from the actor's perspective.

10

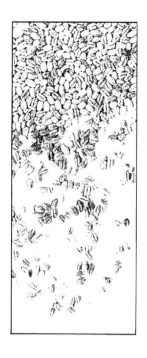

Decision Analysis in Nutrition Studies

Sutti Ortiz

As with Appadurai's contribution, Sutti Ortiz focuses on the way in which people come to do one thing rather than another. But she discusses a different approach, one that looks at the processes by which people decide how to acquire, prepare, and distribute their food. Given the almost complete absence of any application of decision analysis in anthropological studies of dietary practices, her contribution is different from those that have preceded it. It does not present a case study, but draws on case studies in the book to discuss in general terms the significance of decision analysis for understanding dietary practices in domestic contexts.

One of the most important aspects of decision analysis is that the searching and detailed inquiry it involves leads to the posing of critical and basic questions that might otherwise go unasked. In looking at the data presented in some of the case studies, Ortiz suggests that even if researchers choose not to use a decision framework, thinking about dietary practices as solutions to problems gives them different and important insights. The very fact that in some situations decision analysis cannot be applied because, for example, resources and possibilities are too unpredictable for actors to evaluate their options, can itself provide further understanding of the bases of people's actions.

This book is concerned throughout with identifying and analyzing the processes that give rise to particular dietary practices and nutritional statuses in domestic units. An integral part of all such processes is people making (or not making) choices and decisions. This final contribution provides a lucid and thorough outline and method of procedure, not available elsewhere, for investigating further the critical issues of decision making.

So many factors bear on the sequence of activities that results in the flow of nutrients from soil to humans that any research effort must be limited in the activities studied and in the kinds of explanations attempted. But highly focused microstudies, if they are to be useful, need to be set in their appropriate macrocontext and must be properly targeted: The activity examined must be central to the determination of what people consume or how people use food. Once it has been established which are the significant activities, and what social groupings are associated with them, the researcher must decide what framework to use to elicit relevant information and to bring it together in the form of a cogent analysis.

There are three frameworks that can be and have often been used for this purpose: theories that specify the interrelations between factors; observations to help us select how factors interrelate; and subjective information and theoretical assumptions about how people decide to acquire, process, and distribute the food they eat. The second framework is that primarily used by most contributors to this book, with the exception of Appadurai's case study (Chapter 9). Appadurai focuses on subjective information and how people come to do one thing rather than another. But having explored decision analysis (and asked many necessarily searching questions), he found it to be inapplicable to the situation he was studying. This chapter considers the decision format: the questions it asks; the insights it produces, even when it is not the framework used; and procedures for carrying it out.

DECISION ANALYSIS

This approach has been used in anthropology most frequently to analyze production patterns (Barlett ed. 1980; Ortiz 1983; Plattner ed. 1975). In food and nutritional anthropology, the importance of studying the decision-making process is recognized (for example, Goode, Curtis, and Theophano 1984; Lieberman 1986; Van Esterik 1984; and Scrimshaw and Cosminsky, and Sharman, among others in this book) but few studies of the *process* have been carried out. The decision format has, of course, a long history of use in economics of the firm and in studies of consumer behavior. Becker (1965) has also urged economists to employ decision analysis to examine the use of time and assets within the household and, in particular, to examine women's time allocation patterns between household jobs and wage-paying jobs. There is a considerable amount of research on this subject—now graced by the title household economics—some of which is relevant to the issues raised in this book.

One of the pertinent questions asked is when and why do women give up the "drudgery" of food preparation to earn cash. Becker's paradigm begs the answer that it must be when the marginal utility of wages is greater than the marginal utility of housework. In anthropology we prefer to leave a wider margin of answers; yet some aspects of the decision format used by economists is of value, and some of the questions they raise are worth pursuing. Murtaugh (1984), for example, asks why people follow certain shopping frequency patterns (a time allocation issue) and why they purchase certain items over others (a time, preference, and resource allocation problem). He does not, however, make the same assumptions about maximization and utility that are part and parcel of Becker's methodology. He has designed his own decision model, which allows him to search for the answers to the above questions and to check for the validity of his answers within a small population sample.

In Chapter 3, Messer also raises some of the same questions, and I would argue that she may have been able to develop her points a bit further if she had conceived her research as a quest for the solutions to decisions. In her study, time is of the essence to her informants. The women had to work outside the home to have enough money to acquire food; yet working curtailed the time they had to prepare food and forced them to rely on buying snacks for the children. In other words, faced with a time allocation problem, they chose a combined meal and snacking strategy instead of only a full meal strategy. Her study has brought forth rich data, and if we now rephrase it as a decision problem we can begin to answer some of the following equally important questions: Who are the women who chose to work outside the home? What income levels do they aspire to? At what income levels would they turn more of their attention to domestic matters or arrange to delegate them to others? At what income levels does eating strategy revert to a heavier reliance on full meals rather than snacking? The answers to these questions require that we understand some of the intricacies of the time–money allocation problem and that we also understand the relative preferences and payoffs of the various food alternatives and strategies for food processing. In fact, Messer alludes to the relevance of the decision analysis format when she explains that "the decision to make tortillas . . . is a very deliberate one and takes into account the drudgery involved" (see Chapter 3). To explain the decision, she would have had to determine the time required to prepare tortillas and the preference for that food item relative to others that require the same time (which implies the same costs) and that involve lower time or cash costs. If she were to repeat the same exercise for women with different incomes, she would be able to begin to answer some of the preceding questions. In Scrimshaw and Cosminsky's study in Chapter 4, decision analysis would have helped to predict whether nutrient intakes in the commensal unit would improve with greater incomes and how much greater incomes would have to be to make a difference in food intake patterns. Decision analysis would help to phrase the questions more precisely and perhaps allow us to give clearer answers to policymakers.

Murtaugh (1984) uses a decision framework to explore which are the variables that most closely affect activity systems related to nutrition and how each variable affects the food intake of shoppers and of those dependent on them for food. He combines observational and decision approaches to gather the data, not only following shoppers through the supermarket but confronting them with decision questions: Why was a particular item chosen? Why was that item preferred to others? He then plots the questions and answers and tries to simulate the questions and information that the shoppers must have sifted through in order to arrive at their choices. The informants' answers are then used to raise the set of choice questions. Decision elements are employed to reveal the determinants of particular nutrient intakes.

Decision analysis allows us to follow particular activities—

shopping, food preparation, food distribution, and so on—and gives us some hints about the systemic conditions that may affect the flow of activities and the output of the activity system (that is, the quantity and quality of food). It allows us to integrate a considerable amount of data and to organize them diagrammatically. It could also help us to elucidate the possible transformation of food habits in time or with changes of opportunities and incomes.

ASSUMPTIONS THAT LIMIT THE USE OF THE DECISION PARADIGM

Decision analysis is not a panacea. It can be applied only to those cases that share the conditions subsumed under the theoretical assumptions of the approach. The first assumption, which is often overlooked, is that the set of events that activates or channels the flow of food is a consequence of actual choices made by the actors. We should be careful not to impute decisions, though we should be equally careful not to disregard them just because they have not been voluntarily verbalized (see Dehavenon 1978 for nonverbalized command decisions). This is, of course, a very fine-line criterion, but if one is careful it is possible to exclude doubtful material from the analysis and avoid imputation of nonexistent decisions.

One should also exclude from the analysis decisions that do not have food preparation as a central concern. It may well be, as Mary Douglas (Douglas and Isherwood 1979; Douglas 1984) points out, that communication is a very important dimension of consumption and that what is acquired, processed, and distributed has more to do with social relations than with food choice. If the kind of food prepared on particular occasions is a peripheral consideration, these occasions should be excluded from the analysis, even if the amounts of food distributed are considerable. Appadurai clearly explains in Chapter 9 why decision analysis cannot be used when choices involve both food and domestic relations. But if food prepared is a central consideration, then we can still make use of decision analysis, integrating the social and ritual parameters as evaluative considerations in the choice of food, time, and money spent. For example, while I would not use decision analysis to understand the levels of consumption at a pig feast in New Guinea, I would use it to consider variations in the food consumed regularly in a ritual Sunday meal, and sometimes even to evaluate the amount of food given as gifts and expected to be received as gifts.

A second assumption that must be kept in mind is that decision analysis can be applied with ease only when the decisions are discrete events—even though the event may be protracted—and when there is a decision maker who consults, gathers information, and then makes a choice. In other words, if we are dealing with events that are the consequence of negotiations and involve a complex process of interactions and give and take, decision analysis becomes too complex and a not very useful tool (Quinn 1975; Davis 1976). The goal of the decision maker also has to remain constant through the process, though it can change from decision to related decision.

Although the decisions should be discrete events, they can be part of a sequence, each one dependent on the outcome of the previous choice. For example, the amount of food purchased often depends on the amount of money left from another purchase, but if this only limits and does not determine the choice then decision analysis is useful. We only have to integrate the impact of other purchases as possible factors affecting the availability of resources. The important issue is that a previous decision to buy a nonfood item does not preempt the choice of what foods to prepare.

Another important assumption is that the decision problem must have a possible solution. The decision maker must have enough information to evaluate options and discriminate between them. It may take some time before he or she can accumulate sufficient information and process it in such a way as to allow for an evaluative judgment and a choice, but that final step must be possible. When not enough information is available to discriminate between options, the decision maker may delay the choice until costs and payoffs are more clearly discernible (Ortiz 1973). In the process the decision maker may passively wait for more information, may actively seek it, may act haphazardly if hunger makes waiting difficult, or may adopt a holding strategy.

For example, if the decision maker is not sure how much money will be received before the next trip to the supermarket, he or she may haphazardly eat what is at hand, may rely on snacking, or may try to determine whether he or she can borrow money, even if not enough to repeat the already established weekly investment in food purchases. Another example is that of a shopper who knows that the price of potatoes is rising and does not have enough of them on hand to feed the family for a week. This particular shopper is likely to buy more potatoes before they become too expensive, but only if it is possible to estimate what losses may be incurred through spoilage. If the rate of spoilage is difficult to determine, the decision will be delayed until either there are no more potatoes on hand or the price becomes so exorbitant that the loss in income will be definitely higher than any conceived spoilage rate. Thus, incomplete information has the effect of delaying decisions or of shifting strategies.

Cash is not the only uncertain resource; food preparation requires time and the labor of a number of individuals. The availability of helpers and the amount of time that the main cook has at her disposal is not always easy to predict. Individuals have complex time schedules that do not necessarily revolve around food preparation. If the time available is too uncertain, it may also lead to erratic use of stored foods and heavy reliance on snacking. The case of women in Mitla discussed by Messer in Chapter 3 is an appropriate example. Women work to make ends meet, but they are then short of time to prepare labor-demanding tortillas. Time availability, furthermore, becomes uncertain when the working woman has several small children who are constantly demanding attention and who often get sick and require more care. If the women do not earn enough money to delegate domestic responsibilities, or do not have a daughter old enough to assume them, then it is difficult for them to be sure that they will have enough time regularly to prepare traditional meals. Faced with this uncertainty, they change their feeding strategy to one that does not require them often to estimate the time they may have to prepare food—they switch to snacking as a hunger-holding strategy. The women of Mitla face uncertain time availability, but this uncertainty is constrained within a narrow range: They still have from 76 percent to 98 percent of their time to devote to domestic activities. Had time availability become more uncertain (that is, fluctuated within a wider range), their feeding behavior might have been more erratic. In either case, it would be hard to predict when they are likely to give out snacks and the total intake of snacks. Yet decision analysis can be used to explain why unpredictable outcomes are likely and when strategies used may change. It cannot explain *how* strategies may change. For that we have to rely on observations such as those carried out by Messer.

Uncertain incomes may also render food-shopping decisions null and careful budgetary allocation nonexistent. Erratic shopping patterns of low-income households, often blamed on lack of responsibility and of knowledge on the part of the head of the household, can instead be accounted for following the argument in the preceding paragraph. If income variation is extreme and predictability hard to determine, shoppers find it difficult to draw up reasonable food budgets and are unlikely to be willing to stick to a minimum diet all the time. When income becomes available, they may splurge on luxury foods instead of carefully spreading it through subsequent weeks, or they may purchase food randomly in response to hunger or demands from dependents without carefully estimating future cash needs. Thus, policymakers should not jump to conclusions about irresponsible welfare clients, and nutrition analysts should research patterns of consumption when incomes are erratic and low.

Perhaps the most important assumption limiting the use of decision analysis is the fourth—that types and amounts of food to be prepared for consumption are evaluated along important discernible dimensions. For example, we can expect shoppers to consider them according to cost, preparation requirements, assumed nutritional values, social significance, personal and cultural tastes, and so on. Once the foods are evaluated, the ones selected will be those that bring highest satisfaction at that point at lowest cost in time and money. This evaluative process may consist of a single complex pondering period where all the information is spread out and considered, or it may be a series of steps whereby each option is evaluated against another single option. When one of the two options is eliminated, a third option is then contrasted against the one chosen (Murtaugh 1984).

For another example, we can examine shopping behavior when various meats are available for purchase. The shopper may first evaluate pork against beef. If pork is preferred, it will then be compared with chicken, and so on. But the process of sequential choice is a bit more complicated and problematic than in this simplified illustration. Shoppers do not choose between beef and pork by the abstract essence of each item, but by a set of qualitative elements implicit in the meats: price, taste, calories, cooking time, and so on. In the sequential procedure the shopper may contrast the beef with the pork first with respect to price, then taste, and in this way go through the whole set of qualitative elements. Or he may first contrast pork and beef with reference to price, then contrast the favored one with the price of chicken, introducing new elements only when the options are not clear.

The assumption that a decision implies solving problems and evaluating options has encouraged investigators to research actual decision strategies and hypothesize about the conditions that determine the type of evaluative format used. Simon (1957) is one of the pioneers in this field. Originally, he suggested that decision makers did not want to solve problems with maximizing solutions but with satisfying solutions. Later, Tversky (1972) gave up using the decision format implied by utility analysis (see Ortiz 1983) and opted for the digital format implied by computer simulations. He not only proposed—as indicated by the example in the preceding paragraph—that decision makers contrast only two options at a time, but that they eliminate options by considering the aspects of each option following set and predictable procedures. This format has been labeled by Tversky (1972) as "elimination by aspects" and is the one favored by Gladwin (1980), and by Murtaugh (1984) with some minor alterations. Since Tversky's seminal suggestions, a number of researchers have suggested other decision-processing systems (Payne 1976; Einhorn and Hogarth 1981; Klayman n.d.). The best summary and review of ongoing research on the subject is to be found in Einhorn and Hogarth (1981), but we clearly need more careful observation of decision processes outside the laboratory.

If the findings of these researchers are correct, then decision analysts are faced with a new problem: the determination of the format most likely to be used by shoppers and food processors in the particular case they want to analyze. Since the format used may affect the selection of the items purchased, if decision analysis is going to be useful we must determine ahead of time both the choice of options and the format to process them. More research still needs to be done on the subject, and anthropologists are in a particularly good position to carry it out. In other words, we cannot just borrow a decision model and apply it, but we must engage in modelling research while gathering data and examining decisions. Hogarth (1975) has suggested that the model used depends on the computational effort required by the format, decision makers prefer to simplify reasoning tasks when possible. Klayman (n.d.) indicates that it varies with the task and Payne (1976) that it varies with task complexity. Furthermore, it seems that decision makers use multiple formats, switching from one to another. Most of these findings are derived from experimental situations and not from observations of natural decision processes (Quinn 1975); hence, though valuable, they are hypothetical models, which should be researched by anthropologists.

Finally, there is one more limitation to the use of decision analysis for the determination of eating patterns and nutrient intakes. How much, for example, a child eats is not always determined by the cook. It may be guided by social rules (as we have seen in many of the contributions to this book) that indicate the amount that each category of person should receive. But it is also the result of bargaining among siblings and among parents and children. This bargaining process may entail some initial decisions, but it more resembles a gaming situation than a decision model format. It is also very complex and difficult to analyze. Thus, some stages in the flow of food may not lend themselves to decision analysis. In these cases it may be too difficult for the analyst to predict outcomes and variations in outcomes at these stages. Another example is the choice of "menus," which may also not lend itself to decision analysis. This may be the case in the "menu negotiations" discussed by Goode, Curtis, and Theophano (1984), although it is not clear from the data presented. For example, if from observation the analyst determines that the amounts of food distributed through complex bargaining procedures is considerable and may affect the intake levels of commensals, then decision analysis is not applicable in estimating changes in diet and food intake.

STEPS AND PROCEDURES

As must be obvious from the preceding section, a considerable amount of background information is required before one proceeds with decision analysis. One must also determine whether the effort is warranted. This is clearly the case when policy recommendations or theoretical considerations require a precise understanding of factorial interrelation or a quantitative understanding of such interrelations.

Background information is necessary to determine which, if any, are the significant commensal units; how much of the food consumed by individuals flows through the commensal unit and does not depend on individual foraging; and which processing activities are the most significant determinants of levels of nutrient intake and equity in the distribution of nutrients. This information will allow the analyst to target the relevant set of activities and the significant unit for study.

But other background information is necessary to articulate microdecision studies with macroissues. Information must be gathered on ecological, economic, and social factors that affect the flow of food and income to commensal units. In Scrimshaw and Cosminsky's chapter on food procurement and illness on a Guatemalan plantation, for example, it is clear that wages and labor market conditions are the major determinants of income, income fluctuations, and consequently of food intakes. These households are so close to marginal survival that food procurement activities are regarded by Scrimshaw and Cosminsky as means of coping with critical and uncertain situations. Thus, in this case, decisions about time allocation are likely to give priority to income over food preparation, and feeding strategies are likely to respond quickly to changes in income patterns.

In this and similar situations, microdecision analysis should focus on what specific income levels, resources, fringe benefits, and amounts of time for domestic activities are necessary—given the structure of the commensal unit, as well as the prevailing social and cultural values—to ensure adequate diets. A less depressing illustration of how macroevents can affect the flow of food resources to a household is Appadurai's discussion in Chapter 9 of the impact of social exchanges on food flows to households and individuals; in fact, social obligations seem to so much affect food availability that he doubts the validity of microdecision study. Though I do not share his pessimism, clearly a decision analyst must integrate the social macrofactors when considering events within the domestic unit that affect processing and distribution of food.

Several general methodological issues have to be considered when gathering the data for a microdecision study. First, the socioculturally significant period for which detailed and systematic food and time allocation data must be gathered needs to be identified. Messer, in Chapter 3 of this book, regrets not having used "the week" as the time unit of analysis so as to systematically include the Sunday meal in her food intake data. Douglas and Nicod (1974) discuss the symbolic significance of menu variations that for the English household culminate in the Sunday "joint." There are also other significant longer food cycles—ceremonial, harvest, and income—that should be considered. Thus, data must be gathered at different critical times of the year for a socioculturally significant time span.

Observational procedures will also affect the analysis. The researchers in this book, for the most part, favored participant observation techniques. These are very useful techniques, particularly for spotting the unverbalized processes that affect food distribution patterns within the commensal unit. But, in the case of decision analysis, it must be accompanied by more intrusive and structured verbal question-and-answer exchanges. The simplest and most direct manner of linking both techniques is to follow the person or persons responsible for food acquisition, preparation, and distribution through their activities, noting actions and requesting explanations for them. The think-aloud participant technique is the one most often used. Murtaugh (1984) partly relies on it, but he also proposes another research approach that makes extensive use of interview and protocol procedures. There are alternative protocols suggested in market research and consumer behavior literature. Whichever one is used must be closely tailored to the situation being studied. Although market research handbooks may give useful hints, anthropologists should never rely on information gathered from questionnaires. The think-aloud participant technique is still the best compromise. This technique, as also in the case of questionnaires, has been criticized for eliciting rationalizations instead of "the" reason for the choice. This may very well be the case, but the rationalizations will reveal the options that decision makers consider and the style of sifting information and evaluating data that they use when considering options. In other words, the think-aloud technique will help the analyst model the decision process appropriately.

The next task is to select the sample of households to be studied. As Davis (1976) cogently indicates, there is a wide range of solutions to the management of income, together with other resources, and diet. These variations are partly related to ethnic and class background, income levels, health, occupation, compatibility of members of the commensal unit, its structure and authority, and dependency stress. Thus, all of these factors must be considered when selecting and stratifying the sample. But equally relevant are the managerial competency, technical proficiency, and individual interests of the central decision makers. Care must be exercised not to select unrepresentative units in a small sample.

Feeding a family is a process that consists of a number of decision steps. In this sense it has the same pattern as other decision processes (Ortiz 1973; Quinn 1975). The analyst must then determine the various decision points or moments that make up the process, their sequential order, and their interrelation. Participant observation is the most useful technique for mapping decision points. Following the buyer, the cook, and the distributor of food in their activities makes it possible to determine the order and frequency of each action. Direct questions when activities are performed will help determine whether the timing is unusual and the result of a reasoned action—Do you shop every market day or every day? Do you cook this meal every time? Do you prefer to shop on Sundays? Which days do you prefer to shop? The information elicited and the events observed can be used to map the decision points and to determine whether food preparation also depends on parallel sets of decision sequences. For example, Palacio discusses in Chapter 6 the separate contributions of men and women to the food stock of the household. Men contribute rice, flour, and sugar from the proceeds of fish sales. How much they give, or whether they give at all, depends on how much they have earned that week. Women also contribute to the food budget to cover other items in the diet. Food acquisition, in this case, does depend on two parallel decision processes, one of which is contingent on the outcome of the other—that is, women may alter some of their purchases if the men's contribution is low.

The decision analyst must also determine when the decisions are made and what factors may precipitate or delay them. For example, Palacio also tells us that in his Garifuna village fish is so central to the diet that women wait to cook, and hence to decide what other items to cook, until the catch arrives. They then run home to prepare the meal. Availability of fish, or knowledge of when it will be available, determines the timing of the major meal of the Garifuna villagers. It also means that the time needed to prepare the meal cannot be known until the fish arrives, and that the decision of what to cook and how to cook it will depend on the time resource available. The definition of decision points and factors that may affect the timing of decisions is thus very important and will determine resources available when food is processed and even the evaluation of resources available. Information on timing and its variations can be elicited from observations. These data must be supplemented by questions about, for example, what is to be cooked tonight, tomorrow, and so on. I have already discussed this problem in an earlier section in reference to Messer's case study of Mitla women, where constant and unpredictable demands on women's time made it difficult for some mothers to set a time aside for several food preparations during the day. Some women did forgo careful domestic scheduling, responding instead to demands and relying on snacks when time for cooking was not available.

The timing of food preparation also responds to social and cultural events. Ceremonial cycles frequently require elaborate food, festivities are often accompanied by food distribution, and social interactions are often accompanied by food exchanges (see Appadurai, and Theophano and Curtis, in this volume). Some of these events are predictable and are taken into account by those responsible for preparing and distributing of food. For example, in some societies visits are often accompanied by gifts of food, which must be reciprocated at the time. Households know more or less which days of the week or with what frequency these exchanges take place and set aside foods from their stores for this purpose. This information is not lost if the analyst is careful in mapping the decision points and in sorting the factors that delay or precipitate them.

But who are the people who make the food purchases and the preparation decisions? Does the same individual make both? What is at stake for them at the time the decision has to be made? Is their status, rather than the well-being of the commensals, what is relevant? Are authority issues at stake (see Shultz and Theophano 1984)? The social characteristics of the decision makers and their position in the commensal unit must be determined, as they clearly affect the decisions taken. Just as important is to examine the structure of the commensal unit (Scott 1976) to add more information about the social context of provisioning decisions.

Once the timing is determined, the analyst should list what options and information are available to decision makers at that particular time. These are the only choices that are and can be evaluated when shopping, cooking, or distributing food. Since only options available and perceived as available at the time of decision making are likely to be considered, studies of the cost (time, labor, and cash, among others) of all options are not useful. Overly detailed time studies are unnecessary. We need only record time required to perform the tasks considered as possible or relevant at the time of decision.

It is also important to realize that information that has been recently acquired is most likely to be clear in the mind of the decision maker (Ortiz 1979). Information acquired in the past and stored may be recalled in slightly altered form. For example, when food gifts have to be reciprocated the amounts are often evaluated so that they are equivalent to what was received. In some societies accounts are kept and can be used as the source of information; in others, that information rests on the recollection of past exchanges. The memory of prepared foods received some time back is colored by the significance of the gift when it was accepted. If it was received during a period of hunger, the gift is likely to have left a strong feeling of well-being, and the quantity received may loom larger than what it was. The return gift may then reflect, not the actual past transfer, but the transformed recall. Evaluations of time and costs required for the preparation of food for ceremonial occasions may suffer similar distortions. The associated benefits (prestige, laudatory comments, and so on) may color the recall of the time and cash expended to the point that individuals may decide to participate again at times they can ill afford to.

In the evaluation, decision makers also consider satisfaction expected: how the food satisfies hunger, tastes, cultural values, social needs, and so on. Thus, background information on the symbolism of food and food gifts is important. A decision analysis must rest on a knowledge of how various foods are classified and what they represent. For example, in Scrimshaw and Cosminsky's Guatemalan case study in Chapter 4 we learn that eggs and cheese have status significance; hence, they are first of all reserved for men (who eat in public), and only if there is enough money will they be purchased for women (who eat in private).

Furthermore, the options the decision makers are likely to consider are not food items, but bundles of food items. For example, they may think that rice is a routine item and that the choice rests with the type of condiment or sauce that may accompany the rice and whether it will be served with or without meat or fish. In other words, what they are selecting are recipes, cultural prescriptions as to how people must be fed. The chapters by Rizvi and by Theophano and Curtis in this book, as well as an earlier article by Goode, Curtis, and Theophano (1984), illustrate how the cultural prescriptions are used and what their sociocultural significance is. These studies, however, do not give us the full story. Cognitive and cultural analyses often fail to clarify how foods are ranked and their relative significance when options conflict. Decision analysis forces us to examine the more subtle aspects of cultural evaluative procedures.

But how can we determine how the options are judged by decision makers? How can one tell when in a given situation tortillas will be preferred to bread or beans? Only research on cognitive processes can help us answer the first question. But two different courses can be followed to answer the second. One procedure is to draw sets of preference scales by asking informants to choose between given quantities of two items. The same question is repeated, varying only the amounts and noting the combinations that informants consider with indifference. The procedure is again repeated, selecting one of the items from the previous list and contrasting it to a new item. It is important to have informants contrast items that they often have to rank against each other, that is, to simulate the realistic options at any one of the decision points. The other procedure is the one that Murtaugh (1984) uses in his study.

The options considered are not just what foods to prepare or how to prepare them, but also how to organize the preparation. In other words, there are also management decisions that have to be made. This was one of the options, for example, implied in Messer's study, an option requiring decisions that were not often easy to make.

Regardless of how careful we are in designing the decision map, in outlining options, and in determining preferences, it is very hard to integrate all relevant, though perhaps tangential, issues. I am referring to the social consequences of food distribution, which in subtle and reactive ways may affect the behavior of those whose responsibility it is to feed others. Food distribution, even within the family, is a transaction with transactional payoffs. Dehavenon (1978) vividly illustrates this process and explains that the payoff is the subordination of some individuals to others. These processes are seldom verbalized and unlikely to be listed as parameters in a choice. Although a decision analysis may clarify some aspects of these bargaining processes, a fuller understanding can only be gained with detailed observational procedures.

To be of use, decision analysis must follow a careful procedure. If the analyst is cognizant of its limitations, the answers to the questions raised will be significant and will raise new sets of questions. But the exercise will be meaningless if no attempt is made to relate it to major issues that determine the flow of goods, time resources, and cash.

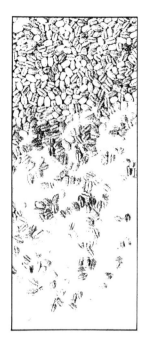

Diet and Domestic Life in Society: Directions for Research and Implications for Policy

Anne Sharman

Janet Theophano

Karen Curtis

Ellen Messer

This book presents a general approach to the study of diet and domestic life in society. At the same time, it represents some of the diversity of theoretical viewpoints characteristic of anthropology and the variety of methods used in small-scale intensive studies. Cumulatively the case studies indicate the need to incorporate the complexity of social situations, including insiders' and outsiders' points of view, into analyses for a well-grounded understanding of the bases of dietary practices and the interrelations between diet, domestic life, and larger-scale social organization. The analyses, in addition, emphasize the need to examine processes giving rise to dietary practices and nutritional status, to carry out studies of what people do over varying periods, to look at the history of social situations and people's circumstances, to try and understand people's experiences and perceptions, to explore how they come to follow one course of action rather than another, and to attempt to find ways of studying how they interact with each other in particular, relevant activity contexts. This final chapter summarizes some topics and methods that require further investigation and development and discusses the policy implications of the approach and data presented.

RESEARCH DIRECTIONS

A central theme in this book is the need to identify the range of domestic groupings and component social relationships in each society under investigation. This directive is so basic that it is a necessary preliminary to any research effort. Equally important are the internal workings of these domestic groupings as they overlap and interrelate. Although all the contributions to this book present some information on this topic, there are still very few studies that focus on detailed analysis of the internal dynamics of domestic units in relation to dietary and health practices. Such studies, albeit difficult and time consuming, are critical for an understanding of the acquisition, allocation, and use of resources; distribution of food; processes of socialization and learning; and, in general terms, decision making.

The content of the workings of domestic units is the practice of daily life: people carrying out activities, interacting, experiencing, learning, deciding, arranging. Only relatively recently have researchers begun to focus on this area in diet-related studies and, together with anthropologists in other fields, begun to develop methods for systematically collecting and analyzing data. Participant observation remains a central method of data collection but is being elaborated and refined in various ways. Social network analysis is being used to systematize and extend data collection to a wider range of relationships and situations, as well as to analyze linkages and interactions within, between, and among domestic units. The observational aspect of participant observation is being enhanced by the more concentrated observational technique of "following," certain categories of people (Messer, Chapter 3; Wilson 1974) and by the use of videotapes in microanalysis (Dehavenon 1978; Johnson 1977, 1980; Shultz and Theophano 1984).

Other researchers have noted that to find out what participants think about what they are doing it is also sometimes necessary to ask them questions during the course of activities, to use a "think aloud" participant technique. A specific form of this kind of method is "contrastive eliciting," used by Murtaugh in studying the decision-making processes of California grocery shoppers (1984). Daily narratives of participants are a way of obtaining a more comprehensive picture of the viewpoints of the people being studied. Life histories and domestic histories provide an approach to looking at the workings of domestic groupings, and at the lives of their members, over longer periods than can be covered by participant observation and personal narratives alone.

In looking at the flow of daily life, it is possible to see some of the ways in which larger-scale organization enters into domestic and local activities and relationships (Vincent 1977), and consequently into dietary practices. The contributions to this book demonstrate that domestic life and the internal dynamics of domestic units are integrally related to systems of social stratification. But more diet-related research is needed in other areas: the material, economic, social, political, and cultural dimensions of social stratification; the interrelations of class, ethnicity, religion, race, and gender in complex systems; the details of wealth, income, and expenditure (consumption) and how these figure in economic and social relationships and in cultural perceptions; the nature and distribution of legal entitlements to food and other resources; the specificity (and thus variability) of the structural and contextual positions of domestic units and their members; and the history of domestic units and their members in relation to changing systems of social stratification. Furthermore in studying the impact of social inequality, it is necessary to look not only at the circumstances of the poor and disadvantaged but also at the situation of those who are more advantageously placed.

Such comparison could contribute to an understanding of the effect of different variables in generating dietary practices and nutritional statuses. Those who are more advantageously placed also may be the employers of those who are poor, and their viewpoints and interests may be significant in the formulation and implementation of policy. More work needs to be done on policies and programs as aspects of large-scale organization and social stratification: as ideology, politics, and business, as well as matters of technical expertise. Thus, for example, in an intensive study at one site of the Special Supplemental Food Program for Women, Infants, and Children (WIC), Sharman (1984) showed how the ongoing conflicts over funding and implementation of the program affected its delivery, and hence the way in which people perceived and used it and its impact. Involved in these conflicts were a diverse array of organizations and individuals representing a range of interests in the program—food companies and industries with their associated interest groups; health and nutrition professionals of different persuasions; advocacy groups; USDA and other government departments with differing responsibilities and concerns; budget officers; WIC administrators and agencies; politicians with contrasting orientations and constituencies; and program participants.

Although work has been done on policies and programs in terms of the interests they represent, and as an aspect of stratification, by other researchers (Friedmann 1982; Taussig 1978), this has not been a significant topic in food and nutritional anthropology, and more investigation is needed. More work also needs to be done on the relation between program implementation and program impact; the interaction between domestic food acquisition and use and food policies and programs; and the dynamics of local-level program implementation (Horowitz 1980; Kennedy and Pinstrup-Andersen 1982; Rogers 1983; Sharman 1984). Participant observation can be extended for studying program formulation and implementation at all levels and used together with different forms of action research.

POLICY IMPLICATIONS

The approach and data presented in this book, together with other studies using a similar orientation, have important implications for policy formulation, implementation, and evaluation.

Formulation

Developing sound food and nutrition policies depends on an understanding of what factors affect diet and nutrition and how, why, to what extent, and in what contexts they do so. Intensive studies using participant observation and case studies are increasingly recognized as one of the potentially most effective ways of answering these questions (Pinstrup-Andersen 1983; Khare 1984). Further, it is increasingly evident that questions of how and why different factors affect diet and nutrition cannot be answered satisfactorily without detailed investigation of domestic life.

What intensive studies seem to suggest, however, is that it is in policy implementation rather than in general policy formulation that domestic organization is of critical importance. Although the bases of dietary practices and nutritional status cannot be fully understood without careful examination of the organization and workings of domestic units, they should *not* be sought *primarily* in the organization of such units (composition, who makes and implements decisions, distribution of food within the domestic unit), in the performance of individuals (skill, health), or in people's beliefs (foods appropriate to particular categories of persons and to particular conditions). Instead, they should be sought in the position of domestic units and their members in society, and the resulting access to resources, patterns of disease and medical care, and opportunities for employment.

It is particularly important to see the situation of women in the context of larger-scale social organization. It is imperative to study women's circumstances and their points of view; to provide resources and services that more equally distribute the burden of their work; and to ensure their rights through legislation. But the problems of women and of men are interrelated and originate not in the characteristics of the domestic group but in the structure of the society (Pala 1977; Burnham 1985). It is, for example, necessary to ask about both the situation of women in poverty and about the employment conditions and opportunities and health of men.

In poor and disadvantaged populations, general policies need to focus on improving the adverse conditions experienced by all categories of people in all situations, not only on helping women and children and on assisting those who are experiencing the worst malnutrition and other consequences of economic deprivation and powerlessness (Gopalan 1984; Khare 1984). Such policies also need to provide for coordinated action in different fields, including food, nutrition, health, and social security (Kennedy and Pinstrup-Andersen 1982). Over the long term, economic policies, including food policies, may be designed to bring about major changes in the distribution of resources and power and in social organization.

Nevertheless, in the short term, political and financial considerations limit what can be achieved. Policies and programs need to be developed for alleviating adverse conditions and for improving the nutrition and health of vulnerable categories of people (particularly women and children) and of those experiencing most hardship. Detailed intensive studies provide information essential as a basis for effective planning of relatively short-term and small-scale local interventions. They suggest that in formulating policy it is necessary to take into account the complexity of the interrelated activities and strategies that people pursue in their attempts to provide adequate resources for themselves and the members of their domestic units and, sometimes, to try to improve their own situation and that of future generations in the long term. If those planning policies and programs look only at outcomes (for example, limited and monotonous diets), they may well underestimate what recipients are capable of doing and misdirect their efforts. They might, for example, overestimate the need for nutrition education and underestimate the need to aid people in their attempts to obtain adequate resources (Rizvi, Chapter 5; Sharman, Chapter 8).

Diet-related activities are often part of detailed adjustments to particular situations, which need to be understood for interventions to be fully effective and not at the same time disruptive in other important areas of people's lives. It is misleading to try to base nutrition and health policies on general, observers' views of the most effective strategies for feeding members of domestic units and for rearing children, and to assume that effective strategies all must have the same style and orientation. The various viewpoints of those for whom policies are being designed need to be taken into account, and recipients need to be involved in the process of formulating, implementing, and evaluating policies and programs at all levels.

Implementation

The analysis of domestic organization and diet-related activities has important implications for planning implementation of general policies and designing specific local programs. Whatever the general policy, if implementation involves domestic units and their members, planning must start from an understanding of the various domestic activity groupings in the area and their interrelationships and internal organization (Messer 1983, 1989; Rogers 1983; Sharman 1970a, 1970b, 1984). Thus, for example, policy to improve the nutrition and health of young children might include provision of food supplements. Whether or not these supplements should be bought or grown (where agriculture or gardening is still an important activity) would depend in part on who controls cash expenditure, who grows and distributes different foodstuffs, and who is responsible for feeding children. Similarly, policies having to choose between the improvement of alternative food crops need to take into account questions of domestic organization and food consumption, as well as those of production; and any educational effort must look carefully at who contributes to decisions about food and health and to their implementation. Usually a more widespread set of relationships is involved than those within the household (Messer 1983, 1989; Sharman 1970a, 1970b, 1984; Theophano and Curtis, Chapter 7).

The contributions to this book also show the often critical significance of informal (as well as more formal) activities for the diet and nutrition of domestic units and their members. It is the informal income-generating and food-acquiring activities of women and children in poor populations that often make it possible for the members of domestic units to survive. Any local implementation of policies and programs must take these activities into account and make sure that they are not inadvertently disrupted without being replaced by some other source of food or income (Rogers 1983). Women's access to resources may depend on secondary rights and informal arrangements and needs to be assured by legal entitlements under conditions of change. Children's participation can be critical and more research needs to be done on how their provisioning activities can be successfully combined with high educational achievement.

Together with informality and complexity, there is often considerable flexibility in the activities and domestic arrangements of poor and disadvantaged people, who frequently depend on short-term sharing and exchange to survive, and who each day must find some way of obtaining basic and necessary resources. Implementation of policies and programs needs to take into account flexibility and variability in domestic arrangements. For example, some rules rigidly specify who may and may not receive and use supplemental foods. This penalizes those who are creative and constructive in using program benefits to improve the nutrition and health of themselves and the members of their domestic units. Flexibility of recipients, their capacity to improvise and to make adjustments, may be important in dealing with the unreliability and shortcomings of program implementation and delivery, as well as with their own inherently precarious situation. Programs often do not allow for variability in domestic arrangements, even where they are designed to be sensitive to cultural variations in food preferences and prohibitions and to individual tastes (Sharman 1984).

Evaluation

The main emphasis in evaluation of food and nutrition policies and programs is usually, and necessarily, on whether they are achieving certain specified, general, and readily measurable objectives, such as increasing intake of certain foodstuffs, improving growth patterns, or reducing anemia in recipients. A secondary concern is often whether the policies and programs being implemented and their methods of delivery are the most effective and efficient way of trying to achieve the specified objectives. Such evaluations, however, are frequently limited in their capacity to assess the impact and functioning of policies and programs, since they look at program "inputs" and program "outputs," but do not look in detail at the processes linking the two (the "black box" approach criticized by such writers as Pinstrup-Andersen 1983 and Rossi and Wright 1984). They do not demonstrate why recipients do or do not show improvement; they do not look at the process of participation and the details of how people use programs, at why programs may be effective for some and not for others, and at the way in which program delivery may directly affect how people use it and thus its impact. The measures used in such evaluations are often also too crude to identify more subtle program benefits, such as the effect on the nutrition and health of people who are not recipients, and are of little help in trying to assess any preventive component in nutrition and health programs.

The approach presented in this book, since it emphasizes the study of processes and the how and why of dietary practices, can be used in exploring the links between program "inputs" and program "outputs," and in tracing the more subtle effects of policies and programs (Sharman 1984). It allows for more detailed analysis, over time, of the processes that link program implementation and impact and of the ways in which food, nutrition, and other interventions enter into, and are used in, the ongoing lives of those whose behavior they are designed to change.

RELEVANCE FOR OTHER DISCIPLINES

Policy formulation, implementation, and evaluation benefit from combining different approaches and different methods of investigation used in a range of disciplines. The emphasis on process and complexity that characterizes the approach presented in this book is sometimes difficult to incorporate into the typically quantitative research designs used by, for example, economists, nutritionists, and health professionals. The challenge for anthropologists using such an approach in working with members of other disciplines is to show:

1. That ethnographic and case-study analysis provides information about and understanding of social processes that cannot be obtained in any other way and that does not lend itself to quantitative analysis
2. How ethnography and case studies can be used to improve the relevance, quality, and accuracy of large-scale surveys: units selected for study, questions to be asked, approaches to asking them (Pelto 1984)
3. How insights derived from ethnography and case study analysis contribute to interpretation of statistical findings
4. How ethnographic and case-study analysis contributes information not obtained by other methods of investigation, which is necessary for ongoing formulation, implementation, and evaluation of food and nutrition policy
5. Ways in which ethnographic and case-study material can be obtained relatively quickly when required for practical purposes

To demonstrate these uses of ethnography and case studies is to make the kind of anthropology presented here accessible to people in other disciplines.

References

Appadurai, A. 1981. "Gastropolitics in Hindu South Asia." *American Ethnologist* 8:494–511.

——. 1984a. "How Moral Is South Asia's Economy? A Review Article." *Journal of Asian Studies* 43:481–97.

——. 1984b. "Wells in Western India: Irrigation and Cooperation in an Agricultural Society." *Expedition* 26:3–14.

——. 1984c. "The Terminology of Measurement in Rural Maharashtra." Manuscript.

——. 1988. "Cookbooks and Cultural Change: The Indian Case." *Comparative Studies in Society and History* 30:3–24.

——, ed. 1986. *The Social Life of Things: Commodities in Cultural Perspective*. Cambridge: Cambridge University Press.

Barlett, P. F., ed. 1980. *Agricultural Decision Making*. New York: Academic.

Becker, G. S. 1965. "A Theory of the Allocation of Time." *The Economic Journal* 75:493–517.

Bertaux, D., ed. 1981. *Biography and Society: The Life History Approach in the Social Sciences*. Beverly Hills, California: Sage.

Bertaux, D., and M. Kohli. 1984. "The Life Story Approach: A Continental View." *Annual Review of Sociology* 10:215–37.

Bourdieu, P. 1977. *Outline of a Theory of Practice*. Cambridge: Cambridge University Press.

Burgess, M. 1976. *Soul to Soul: A Vegetarian Soul Food Cookbook*. Santa Barbara, California: Woodbridge.

Burkill, I. H. 1966. *A Dictionary of the Economic Products of the Malay Peninsula*. Kuala Lumpur: Ministry of Agriculture and Cooperatives.

Burnham, L. 1985. "Has Poverty Been Feminized in Black America?" *The Black Scholar* 16:14–24.

Chambers, R., R. Longhurst, and A. Pacey, eds. 1981. *Seasonal Dimensions to Rural Poverty*. London: Frances Pinter.

Chaney, E. M. 1985. *Migration from the Caribbean Region: Determinants and Effects of Current Movements*. Washington, D.C.: Georgetown University, Center for Immigration Policy and Refugee Assistance.

Cicourel, A. 1964. *Method and Measurement in Sociology*. New York: Free Press.

Cosminsky, S. 1987. "Women and Health Care on a Guatemalan Plantation." *Social Science and Medicine* 25 (10):1163–73.

Cosminsky, S., and M. Scrimshaw. 1980. "Medical Pluralism on a Guatemalan Plantation." *Social Science and Medicine* 14B:267–78.

———. 1981. "Sex Roles and Subsistence: A Comparative Analysis of Three Central American Communities." In *Sex Roles and Social Change in Native Lower Central American Societies*, ed. C. Loveland and F. Loveland, 44–69. Urbana: University of Illinois Press.

Curtis, K. 1983. *"I Can Never Go Anywhere Empty Handed": Food Exchange and Reciprocity in an Italian American Community*. Ann Arbor, Michigan: University Microfilms.

Curtis, K., and J. Theophano. 1981. "Two Women in the Field." Manuscript.

Darden, N. J., and C. Darden. 1978. *Spoonbread and Strawberry Wine*. New York: Fawcett Crest.

Davis, H. L. 1976. "Decision Making in Households." *Journal of Consumer Research* 2:241–60.

Dehavenon, A. L. 1978. "Superordinate Behavior in Urban Homes: A Video Analysis of Request-Compliance and Food Control Behavior in Two Black and Two White Families Living in New York City." Ph.D. dissertation, Columbia University.

Dengler, I. C. 1979. "Soul Food: That's What I Like." *Foodtalk* 2:1, 2, 8.

Dewalt, K. M. 1983. "Income and Dietary Adequacy in an Agricultural Community." *Social Science and Medicine* 17:1877–86.

Dewalt, K. M., P. B. Kelly, and G. H. Pelto. 1980. "Nutritional Correlates of Economic Microdifferentiation in a Highland Mexican Community." In *Nutritional Anthropology*, ed. N. W. Jerome, R. F. Kandel, and G. H. Pelto, 205–22. New York: Redgrave.

di Leonardo, M. 1984. *The Varieties of Ethnic Experience: Kinship, Class, and Gender Among California Italian-Americans.* Ithaca, New York: Cornell University Press.

Douglas, M. 1978. *Cultural Bias.* London: Royal Anthropological Institute.

———, ed. 1984. *Food in the Social Order.* New York: Russell Sage Foundation.

Douglas, M., and J. Gross. 1981. "Food and Culture: Measuring the Intricacy of Rule Systems." *Social Science Information* 20:1–35.

Douglas, M., and B. Isherwood. 1979. *The World of Goods.* New York: Basic.

Douglas, M., and M. Nicod. 1974. "Taking the Biscuit: The Structure of British Meals." *New Society* 30:744–47.

Dunn, F. L. 1975. *Rain-Forest Collectors and Traders: A Study of Resource Utilization in Modern and Ancient Malaya.* Monograph No. 5, Malaysian Branch of the Royal Asiatic Society.

Eide, W. B. 1982. "The Nutrition Educator's Role in Access to Food: From Individual Orientation to Social Orientation." *Journal of Nutrition Education* 14:14–17.

Einhorn, H. J., and R. M. Hogarth. 1981. "Behavioral Decision Theory: Processes of Judgment and Choice." *Annual Review of Psychology* 2:53–88.

Erasmus, C. J. 1980. "Comment on Wanda Minge-Klevana: Does Labor Time Decrease with Industrialization? A Survey of Time-Allocation Studies." *Current Anthropology* 21:289–91.

Firth, Raymond. [1936] 1957. *We, the Tikopia.* London: Allen and Unwin.

———. [1946] 1966. *Malay Fishermen: Their Peasant Economy.* New York: Norton.

Firth, Rosemary. [1943] 1966. *Housekeeping Among Malay Peasants.* London: Athlone.

Friedmann, H. 1982. "The Political Economy of Food: The Rise and Fall of the Postwar International Food Order." In *Marxist Inquiries: Studies of Labor, Class, and States*, ed. M. Buroway and T. Skocpol, 248–86. *American Journal of Sociology* 88, Supplement.

Geertz, C. 1973. *The Interpretation of Cultures.* New York: Basic.

Gilbert, D. 1976. "A Dietary Survey of Guatemalan Women on the Finca San Luis." Department of Nutrition, M.I.T. Manuscript.

Gladwin, C. 1980. "A Theory of Real Life Choice: Applications to Agricultural Decisions." In *Agricultural Decision Making,* ed. P. Barlett, 45–85. New York: Academic.

Gladwin, H., and M. Murtaugh. 1980. "The Attentive-Preattentive Distinction in Agricultural Decision Making." In *Agricultural Decision Making,* ed. P. F. Barlett, 115–36. New York: Academic.

Gluckman, M. 1961. "Ethnographic Data in British Social Anthropology." *Sociological Review* 9:5–17.

Goode, J., K. Curtis, and J. Theophano. 1984. "Meal Formats, Meal Cycles, and Menu Negotiations in the Maintenance of an Italian-American Community." In *Food in the Social Order,* ed. M. Douglas, 143–218. New York: Russell Sage Foundation.

Goody, E. 1978. "Delegation of Parental Roles in West Indies and Africa." In *The Extended Family in Black Societies,* ed. D. B. Shimkin, E. M. Shimkin, and D. A. Frate, 447–84. The Hague: Mouton.

Gopalan, C. 1984. "The Nutrition Policy of Brinkmanship." *ICAF Occasional Report* 3:6–7.

Gross, D., and B. Underwood. 1971. "Technological Change and Caloric Costs: Sisal Agriculture in Northwestern Brazil." *American Anthropologist* 73:725–40.

Guatemala–A.I.D. 1977. "Extension of Health Services to Finca Workers." Guatemala Health Sector Assessment, Annex 5.7. Academic de Ciencias Medicas and U.S.A.I.D., Guatemala. Manuscript.

Gulati, L. 1981. *Profiles in Female Poverty: A Study of Five Poor Working Women in Kerala.* Oxford: Pergamon.

Harrison, B. 1979. "Welfare Payments and the Reproduction of Low-Wage Workers and Secondary Jobs." *The Review of Radical Political Economics* 11:1–16.

Hertzler, A. A., and C. Owen. 1976. "Sociologic Study of Food Habits: A Review. I., Diversity in Diet and Scalogram Analysis." *Journal of the American Dietetic Association* 69:377–81.

Hogarth, R. M. 1975. "Cognitive Processes and the Assessment of Subjective Probability Distributions." *Journal of the American Statistical Association* 70:271–94.

Horowitz, G. 1980. "Intra-Family Distribution of Food and Other Resources." Report for the Nutrition Economics Group, U.S.A.I.D., Washington, D.C.

Jerome, N. W. 1980. "Diet and Acculturation: The Case of Black American In-Migrants." In *Nutritional Anthropology*, ed. N. W. Jerome, R. F. Kandel, and G. H. Pelto, 275–325. New York: Redgrave.

Johnson, O. R. 1977. *Domestic Organization and Interpersonal Relations Among the Machiguenga Indians of the Peruvian Amazon*. Ann Arbor, Michigan: University Microfilms.

———. 1980. "The Social Context of Intimacy and Avoidance: A Videotape Study of Machiguenga Meals." *Ethnology* 19:353–66.

Kennedy, E., and P. Pinstrup-Andersen. 1982. *Nutrition-Related Policies and Programs: Past Performance and Research Needs*. Washington, D.C.: International Food Policy Research Institute.

Khare, R. S. 1976a. *The Hindu Hearth and Home*. New Delhi: Vikas.

———. 1976b. *Culture and Reality: Essays on the Hindu System of Managing Foods*. Simla: Indian Institute of Advanced Study.

———. 1984. "Anthropology and Nutrition Policy Issues: Some Comments." *I.C.A.F. Occasional Report* 3:7.

Klayman, J. n.d. "Simulation of Six Decision Strategies: Comparison of Search Patterns, Processing Characteristics, and Response to Task Complexity." University of Chicago, Center for Decision Research. Manuscript.

Kolasa, K. M. 1974. *Foodways of Selected Mothers and Their Adult Daughters in Upper East Tennessee*. Ann Arbor, Michigan: University Microfilms.

Laderman, C. C. 1979. *Conceptions and Preconceptions: Childbirth and Nutrition in Rural Malaysia*. Ann Arbor, Michigan: University Microfilms.

———. 1981. "Symbolic and Empirical Reality: A New Approach to the Analysis of Food Avoidances." *American Ethnologist* 8:468–93.

———. 1983. *Wives and Midwives: Childbirth and Nutrition in Rural Malaysia*. Berkeley: University of California Press.

———. 1984. "Food Ideology and Eating Behavior: Contributions from Malay Studies." *Social Science and Medicine* 19:547–59.

Lamphere, L. 1974. "Strategies, Cooperation, and Conflict Among Women in Domestic Groups." In *Women, Culture, and Society*, ed. M. Z. Rosaldo and L. Lamphere, 97–112. Stanford, California: Stanford University Press.

Lewin, K. 1943. "Forces Behind Food Habits and Methods of Change." In *The Problem of Changing Food Habits*. National Research Council Bulletin 108:35–65. Washington, D.C.: National Academy of Sciences–National Research Council.

Lieberman, L. S. 1986. "Nutritional Anthropology at the Household Level." In *Training Manual in Nutritional Anthropology*, ed. S. A. Quandt and C. Ritenbaugh. Washington, D.C.: American Anthropological Association.

Lindenbaum, S. 1986. "Rice and Wheat: The Meaning of Food in Bangladesh." In *Food, Society, and Culture*, ed. R. S. Khare and M. A. Rao. Durham, North Carolina: Carolina Academic.

Lord, D. G. 1975. *Money Order Economy: Remittances in the Island of Utila*. Ann Arbor, Michigan: University Microfilms.

Marchione, T. J. 1980. "Factors Associated with Malnutrition in the Children of Western Jamaica." In *Nutritional Anthropology*, ed. N. W. Jerome, R. F. Kandel, and G. H. Pelto, 222–74. New York: Redgrave.

———. 1981. "Child Nutrition and Dietary Diversity Within the Family." *Food and Nutrition Bulletin* 3:10–14.

Marcus, G. E., and D. Cushman. 1982. "Ethnographies as Texts." *Annual Review of Anthropology* 11:25–69.

Marriott, M. 1968. "Caste Ranking and Food Transactions: A Matrix Analysis." In *Structure and Change in Indian Society*, ed. M. Singer and B. S. Cohn, 133–71. Chicago: Aldine.

———. 1976. "Hindu Transactions: Diversity Without Dualism." In *Transaction and Meaning*, ed. B. Kapferer, 109–42. Philadelphia: Institute for the Study of Human Issues.

Massard, J. 1983. *Nous Gens de Ganchong: Environnement et Echanges dans un Village Malais*. Paris: Editions du Centre National de la Recherche Scientifique.

Mead, M. 1943. "The Problem of Changing Food Habits." In *The Problem of Changing Food Habits*. National Research Council Bulletin 108:20–31. Washington, D.C.: National Academy of Sciences–National Research Council.

———. 1949. "Cultural Patterning of Nutritionally Relevant Behavior." *Journal of the American Dietetic Association* 25:677–80.

Messer, E. 1983. "The Household Focus in Nutritional Anthropology: An Overview." *Food and Nutrition Bulletin* 5:2–12.

———. 1984a. "Sociocultural Aspects of Nutrient Intake and Behavioral Responses to Nutrition." In *Nutrition and Behavior*, ed. J. Galler. New York: Plenum.

———. 1984b. "Anthropological Perspectives on Diet." *Annual Reviews in Anthropology* 13:205–49.

————. 1986. "Some Like It Sweet: Estimating Sweetness Preferences and Sucrose Intakes from Ethnographic and Experimental Data." *American Anthropologist* 88:637–47.

————. 1989. "The Relevance of Time Allocation Studies for Nutritional Anthropology." In *Methods in Nutritional Anthropology*, ed. G. H. Pelto, P. Pelto, and E. Messer. Tokyo: United Nations University.

Miller, B. D. 1981. *The Endangered Sex: Neglect of Female Children in Rural North India*. Ithaca, New York: Cornell University Press.

Mitchell, J. C. 1983. "Case and Situation Analysis." *Sociological Review* 31: 187–211.

Montgomery, E. 1978. "Anthropological Contributions to the Study of Food-Related Cultural Variability." In *Progress in Human Nutrition*, vol. 2, ed. S. Margen and R. A. Ogar, 42–56. Westport, Connecticut: Avi.

Muhammad, E. 1967, 1972. *How to Eat to Live: Books 1 and 2*. Chicago: Muhammad's Temple of Islam No. 2.

Mullings, L. 1978. "Ethnicity and Stratification in the Urban United States." *Annals of the New York Academy of Sciences*, 318:10–22.

Murtaugh, M. 1984. "Model of Grocery Shopping Decision Process Based on Verbal Protocol Data." *Human Organization* 43:243–51.

Nadel, S. F. 1956. *Theory of Social Structure*. London: Cohen & West.

Nag, M. J., B. White, and R. C. Peet. 1978. "An Anthropological Approach to the Study of the Economic Value of Children in Java and Nepal." *Current Anthropology* 19:293–306.

Ortiz, S. 1973. *Uncertainties in Peasant Farming*. London: Athlone.

————. 1979. "Expectations and Forecasts in the Face of Uncertainty." *Man* 14:64–80.

————. 1983. "What Is Decision Analysis About?" In *Economic Anthropology*, ed. S. Ortiz, 249–97. Lanham, Maryland: University Press of America.

Ortner, S. 1978. *Sherpas Through Their Rituals*. Cambridge: Cambridge University Press.

————. 1984. "Theory in Anthropology Since the Sixties." In *Comparative Studies in Society and History* 26:126-66.

Pala, A. O. 1977. "Definitions of Women and Development: An African Perspective." In *Women and National Development: The Complexities of Change*, Wellesley Editorial Committee, 9–13. Chicago: University of Chicago Press.

Palacio, J. O. 1982. *Food and Social Relations in a Garifuna Village*. Ann Arbor, Michigan: University Microfilms.

———. 1983. "Food and Body in Garifuna Belief Systems." *Cajanus* 16: 149–60.

Papanek, H. 1979. "Family Status Production: The "Work" and "Non-Work" of Women." *Signs* 4:775–81.

———. 1984. "False Specialization and the Purdah of Scholarship: A Review Article." *Journal of Asian Studies*, 44:127–48.

Payne, J. W. 1976. "Task Complexity and Contingent Processing in Decision Making: An Information Search and Protocol Analysis." *Organizational Behavior and Human Performance* 16:366–87.

Peck, E. 1970. "Nutrition and Health Status on a Guatemalan Costal Finca." INCAP, Guatemala. Manuscript.

Pelto, G. H. 1983. "Intra-Household Food Distribution Patterns." *Proceedings of the Western Hemisphere Nutrition Congress* 7, August.

———. 1984. "Ethnographic Studies of the Effects of Food Availability and Infant Feeding Practices." *Food and Nutrition Bulletin* 6:33–43.

Perry, H. 1978. "The Metonymic Definition of the Female and the Concept of Honour Among Italian Immigrant Families in Toronto." In *The Italian Immigrant Woman in North America*, ed. B. Caroli, R. Harney, and L. Tomasi. Toronto: Multicultural History Society of Ontario.

Pinstrup-Andersen, P. 1983. "Estimating the Nutritional Impact of Food Policies: A Note on the Analytical Approach." *Food and Nutrition Bulletin* 5:16–21.

Plattner, S., ed. 1975. *Formal Methods in Economic Anthropology*. Washington, D.C.: American Anthropological Association Special Publication No. 4.

Quinn, N. 1975. "Decision Models of Social Structure." *American Ethnologist* 2:19–47.

Rapp, R. 1978. "Family and Class in Contemporary America: Notes Toward an Understanding of Ideology." *Science and Society* 42:278–300.

Richards, A. I. 1939. *Land, Labour, and Diet in Northern Rhodesia*. London: Routledge.

Rizvi, N. 1979. *Rural and Urban Food Behavior in Bangladesh: An Anthropological Perspective to the Problem of Malnutrition*. Ann Arbor, Michigan: University Microfilms.

———. 1983. "Effects of Food Policy on Intra-Household Food Distribution in Bangladesh." *Food and Nutrition Bulletin* 5:30–34.

————. 1986. "Food Categories in Bangladesh, and Its Relationship to Food Beliefs and Practices of Vulnerable Groups." In *Food, Society, and Culture* ed. R. S. Khare and M. S. A. Rao. Durham, North Carolina: Carolina Academic.

Rogers, B. L. 1983. "The Internal Dynamics of Households: A Critical Factor in Development Policy." Tufts University School of Nutrition. Report Prepared for U.S.A.I.D./P.P.C./P.D.P.R./H.R.

Rossi, P. H., and J. D. Wright. 1984. Evaluation Research and Assessment. *Annual Reviews in Sociology* 10:331–52.

Rutz, H. J., and B. S. Orlove, eds. 1989. *The Social Economy of Consumption.* Lanham, Maryland: University Press of America.

Sahlins, M. 1965. "On the Sociology of Primitive Exchange." In *The Relevance of Models for Social Anthropology*, ed. M. Banton. New York: Praeger.

Schutz, A. 1970. *Reflections on the Problem of Relevance.* New Haven, Connecticut: Yale University Press.

Scott, R. 1976. *The Female Consumer.* New York: Halsted.

Shack, W. 1976. "A Taste of Soul." *New Society* 37:127.

Sharma, U. 1980. *Women, Work, and Property in North-West India.* London: Tavistock.

Sharman, A. 1970a. "Social and Economic Aspects of Nutrition in Padhola, Bukedi District, Uganda." Ph.D. dissertation, University of London.

————. 1970b. "Nutrition and Social Planning." *Journal of Development Studies* 6:77–91.

————. 1984. "Supplemental Food Programs and Domestic Resource Allocation: A Case from the WIC Program." Manuscript.

Shultz, J., and J. Theophano. 1984. "Locating Learning in Social Interaction at Meal Times." Manuscript.

Simon, H. A. 1957. *Models of Man, Social and Rational.* New York: Wiley.

Stack, C. B. 1974. *All Our Kin: Strategies for Survival in a Black Community.* New York: Harper-Colophon.

Stone, L. 1978. "Food Symbolism in Hindu Nepal." *Contributions to Nepalese Studies* 6:47–65.

Taussig, M. 1978. "Nutrition, Development, and Foreign Aid: A Case Study of U.S. Directed Health Care in a Colombian Plantation Zone." *International Journal of Health Services* 8:101–21.

Theophano, J. S. 1982. *"It's Really Tomato Sauce but We Call It Gravy": A Study of Food and Women's Work Among Italian-American Families.* Ann Arbor, Michigan: University Microfilms.

Tversky, A. 1972. "Elimination by Aspects: A Theory of Choice." *Psychological Review* 79:281–99.

U.S. Department of Agriculture. 1978. *Food Consumption Prices and Expenditures.* Supplement for Agriculture and Economics Report No. 138. Washington, D.C.: U.S. Department of Agriculture.

Valverde, V. 1985. "Nutrition and Health Consequences of Seasonal Fluctuations in Household Food Availability." Paper presented at the workshop, Impact of Agriculture and Food Supply Policies on Nutrition and Health Status, Bellagio, Italy.

Van Esterik, P. 1984. *Intra-Family Food Distribution: Its Relevance for Maternal and Child Nutrition.* Cornell Nutritional Surveillance Program, Working Paper Series, No. 31. Ithaca, New York: Cornell University.

Vincent, J. 1977. "Agrarian Society as Organized Flow: Processes of Development Past and Present." *Peasant Studies* 6:56–65.

Wallman, S. 1984. *Eight London Households.* London: Tavistock.

Watson, J. L. 1977. "The Chinese: Hong Kong Villagers in the British Catering Trade." In *Between Two Cultures: Migrants and Minorities in Britain*, ed. J. L. Watson, 181–213. Oxford: Basil Blackwell.

Whitehead, T. L. 1978. "Industrialization, Social Networks, and Food Flow: Survival Strategies in a Jamaican Sugartown." Paper presented to the Symposium on Anthropology, Nutrition, and Policy Planning, International Congress of Union of Anthropological and Ethnological Sciences, New Delhi.

———. 1984. "Sociocultural Dynamics and Food Habits in a Southern Community." In *Food in the Social Order*, ed. M. Douglas, 97–142. New York: Russell Sage Foundation.

Wilks, R. R., ed. 1989. *The Household Economy.* Boulder, Colorado: Westview.

Wilson, C. S. 1970. *Food Beliefs and Practices of Malay Fishermen: An Ethnographic Study of Diet on the East Coast of Malaya.* Ann Arbor, Michigan: University Microfilms.

———. 1974. "Child Following: A Technique for Learning Food and Nutrient Intakes." *Journal of Tropical Pediatrics and Environmental Child Health* 20:9–14.

Wolff, R. 1965. "The Meanings of Food." *Journal of Tropical and Geographical Medicine* 1:45–51.

The Contributors

Arjun Appadurai (Ph.D. University of Chicago, 1976) is a professor of anthropology at the University of Pennsylvania. He has conducted fieldwork in rural western and in urban south India and is currently engaged in a study of contemporary public culture in that country. He is author of *Worship and Conflict Under Colonial Rule* (Cambridge: Cambridge University Press, 1981) and editor of *The Social Life of Things: Commodities in Cultural Perspective* (Cambridge: Cambridge University Press, 1986).

Sheila Cosminsky (Ph.D. Brandeis University, 1972) is an associate professor of anthropology at Rutgers University, Camden Campus. She has done fieldwork in Guatemala, Belize, Kenya, and Zimbabwe in areas relating to maternal and child health, nutrition, and ethnomedicine. Her publications include *Traditional Medicine: An Annotated Bibliography* (New York: Garland Press, 1982, with I. Harrison) and numerous articles on medical and nutritional anthropology.

Karen Curtis (Ph.D. Temple University, 1984) is an associate policy scientist and assistant professor in the College of Urban Affairs and Public Policy, University of Delaware. She is an urban applied anthropologist and has done research on social networks and food exchange and work on evaluation of a variety of social programs. She is active in local and national associations of practicing anthropologists and of urban anthropologists. She has published on the anthropology of food, employment and training, special education, and economic development.

Carol Laderman (Ph.D. Columbia University, 1979) is a professor of anthropology and chairperson of the Department of Anthropology at the City College, City University of New York. She edited *Techniques of Healing in Southeast Asia*, which appeared as a special issue of *Social Science and Medicine* (vol. 27, no. 8, 1988), and she has published two books: *Wives and Midwives: Childbirth and Nutrition in Rural Malaysia* (Berkeley: University of California Press, 1983) and *Taming the Wind of Desire: Psychology, Medicine and Aesthetics in Malay Shamanistic Performance* (Berkeley: University of California Press, forthcoming).

Ellen Messer (Ph.D. University of Michigan, 1975) is an anthropologist trained at Harvard and Michigan. She carried out fieldwork on ethnobotany, socioeconomics, and food consumption in two towns in Oaxaca, Mexico, between 1971 and 1981. She is past president of the Council on Nutritional Anthropology of the American Anthropological Association and an associate professor in the Alan Shawn Feinstein World Hunger Program, Brown University. She is also a Visiting Scholar in the International Food and Nutrition Program at MIT.

Sutti Ortiz (Ph.D. University of London, 1963) is an associate professor of anthropology, Boston University. In her research she has focused on economic organization and economic development. She has paid particular attention to the study of time and resource allocations, using a decision-analysis perspective. She has written as well on marketing systems, resettlement of populations in frontier areas, and at present, on labor markets in commercial agriculture.

Joseph Palacio (Ph.D. University of California, Berkeley, 1982) is Resident Tutor in the School of Continuing Studies of the University of the West Indies in Belize. His research interests include archaeology of the Mesoamerican area and social anthropology of Central America and the Caribbean. He has published articles on migration, food studies, and community development, as well as on archaeology.

Najma Rizvi (Ph.D. University of California, Los Angeles, 1979) is an anthropologist working in the Department of Pediatrics at the University of Iowa. Her major areas of professional interest are rural and urban food behavior, maternal-child health and nutrition, illness-management patterns, and the role of women in the household decision-making process. She has done fieldwork in Bangladesh, Pakistan, and the United States, dealing with issues that have policy implications.

Mary Scrimshaw is Commissioner for the Western Hemisphere for the International Commission on Anthropology and Food, IUAES. After graduate work in genetics, she studied anthropology at the University of San Carlos, Guatemala, and at Brandeis University. She has worked with market women in Guatemala and the Dominican Republic and women tea pickers in Java, and she has carried out a longitudinal study of fertility, food procurement, and health care in Guatemala. She has held offices on the Council on Nutritional Anthropology of the American Anthropological Association.

Anne Sharman (Ph.D. University of London, 1970) is a nutrition manager on the WIC Program in Philadelphia. From 1977 to 1983 she was a senior research associate at the Institute for the Study of Human Issues, Philadelphia, and from 1969 to 1978 held a teaching position at the University of East Anglia. As an anthropologist she has done work in Uganda and Philadelphia on diet and nutrition and has published in this field.

Janet Theophano (Ph.D. University of Pennsylvania, 1982) is assistant dean and assistant director of the College of General Studies at the University of Pennsylvania. She is also adjunct assistant professor of folklore and director of the Social Gerontology Program. She has done fieldwork on food patterns in Italian-American and Greek-American communities, as well as work on nutritional assessment in an inner-city Puerto Rican and black community.

Index

Activities: interrelation of dietary, domestic, and other, 5–6, 8–10, 35–36, 41–48, 63, 96–98, 155–56, 183–87, 217–29, 244–45, 255–56; social analysis and, 5–6, 8–10, 235, 237–38. *See also* Time allocation and activity patterns

Activity groupings, 9–10, 16, 25, 95, 96–97, 130–31, 137, 159–65, 166, 169, 228, 231n, 244, 259–60

African Americans (in a northeastern city): case studies of, 183–93; diet of, 178–80, 187–93; life histories of, 181–87

Age, food distribution and, 48–49, 105–6, 111, 114–15, 217. *See also* Children; Elderly, the; Men; Women

Agriculture, 18–19, 38, 67, 94–95, 96–97, 128, 130–31, 210–11

Alcohol and alcoholism, 45, 65, 74, 77, 78, 80, 87, 142–43

Animal husbandry, 17, 38, 69, 85

Anthropology: food and nutritional, 4–5, 62, 92, 206, 235; food and nutrition policy and, 5, 10, 92, 118; fields of study in, 255; theoretical traditions in, 6, 120, 148–49, 254

Appadurai, A., 6, 206, 208, 209, 210, 222, 234, 235, 238, 245, 248

Bangladesh: food and nutrition policy in, 92, 116–18; food ideology and diet in, 101–7; intrahousehold food distribution in, 105–6, 107, 111–15; interhousehold food distribution in, 107–11; rural, 93–97, 99–100, 110–11; socioeconomic factors and diet in, 107–11; urban, 97–98, 100

277